TARA MILLER

Wall Pilates

28 Day Challenge Series

First edition

This book was professionally typeset on Reedsy.
Find out more at reedsy.com

Contents

Introduction

Congratulations on wanting a more firm and toned body! Wall pilates is a great way to begin your weight loss journey. You can add variety and challenge by using wall pilates if you are continuing your health and weight loss journey as well!

Starting a Fitness Journey

As with beginning any fitness journey, you should check with your doctor to make sure you are healthy to begin exercising.

What is Wall Pilates

As the name implies, wall pilates is an offshoot of traditional pilates. While conventional pilates requires the use of a mat and specialized equipment, wall pilates harnesses the use of the wall as a tool for enhancing stability and alignment and is easily done at home without expensive equipment or a pilates studio membership.

Benefits of Practicing Wall Pilates

The use of the wall provides enhanced stability and alignment which connects the body with its sense of gravity and awareness of posture. The movements activate your core and strengthen your abdomen, pelvis, and lower back. As your journey continues, you will notice improved flexibility and range of motion due to the elongation of muscles, tendons, and ligaments by continuously stretching and moving. Pilates traditionally incorporates mindfulness and body awareness, but with the incorporation of the wall, it can allow a deeper mind and body connection by allowing sensory feedback which helps you to refine your movements. One of my favorite reasons for practicing wall pilates is the ease of versatility and accessibility. Very little equipment is required which makes it applicable to those of all fitness levels and adaptable for different needs and goals.

Motivation and Accountability

In order to stay accountable, make sure to schedule your wall pilates workouts into your weekly routine. Block out a time each day for your workout. Just like any other important appointment, your wall pilates workout should be non-negotiable. To remain consistent, try to aim for the same time each day, but don't let a missed scheduled time stop you from fitting it in later the same day.

About Your Diet

While you are focusing on your health and fitness, be sure to maintain a balanced and nutritious diet. I'm not going to go into a whole dieting plan in this book but do your best to support your goals by trying to stay within a few guidelines. Make sure to stay hydrated throughout your fitness journey. Hydration promotes overall well-being, digestion, and proper muscle function. Try to focus on eating whole foods. They will provide the essential nutrients a hard-working body needs for optimal performance as well as essential vitamins, minerals, and antioxidants. A whole foods diet consists of fruits, vegetables, whole grains, lean proteins, and healthy fats. Lean protein supports muscle repair and growth. Some of these include chicken, turkey, fish, tofu, tempeh, legumes, and some lower-fat dairy products. Whole grains and complex carbohydrates fuel the body and replenish glycogen stores. Examples include brown rice, oats, quinoa, whole wheat, and also starchy vegetables like potatoes, sweet potatoes, squash, and legumes such as beans and lentils. If you are trying to lose fat you will want to go easy on the fats even if they are healthy fats. Some of these include avocados, nuts, seeds, oils, and fatty fish. Salmon and mackerel are some examples of fatty fish.

Remember to eat your balanced meals and snacks regularly throughout the day. Eating at regular intervals will help to prevent overeating and sustain your energy levels. Some balanced meal examples include a protein fruit smoothie, whole grain turkey sandwich, grilled chicken or tempeh and vegetable bowl with rice or quinoa, grilled chicken or tofu, and veggie on lavash wrap. Good examples of snacks include an apple with natural peanut butter, banana and almond butter, avocado on whole grain toast, or yogurt with fruit. Don't make eating healthy complex and difficult. Pick out a few favorite meals and eat them throughout the week, then pick out a few different ones for the next week to prevent food boredom.

One more important tip when dieting, if you find yourself craving something even after drinking 8 oz. of water and waiting 10-15 minutes go ahead and enjoy a treat or indulgence - in moderation. Remember that it's essential to fuel your body with nutritious foods but you can have a balanced diet and have a small treat every once in a while during your journey. This makes dieting more sustainable.

List of Equipment

The only thing necessary is the wall but here is a list of optional items to make your experience challenging and effective as well as comfortable. Some of the exercises suggest using a resistance band, but it is not necessary. Use one if you would like to make the workout more difficult or advanced.

- Wall - The most important thing you need for wall pilates is a wall. It should be a sturdy flat wall that is away from any protrusions or objects.
- Exercise mat - An exercise mat is not required but I recommend one to prevent slipping and sliding around and also to cushion and support your back.
- Resistance band - Also not a requirement, a resistance band can add another level of difficulty and intensity to the workouts.
- Water - Make sure to drink plenty of water to keep hydrated.
- Towel - You may want a towel to wipe away sweat and keep your exercise area dry.
- Clothing - Be sure to wear clothing that allows for a full range of motion.
- Footwear - I recommend bare feet, but feel free to wear gripping socks or if needed, light flexible shoes.
- Mirror - A mirror can benefit you by allowing you to see your form and alignment.
- Journal - Use a journal, notebook, or calendar to track your fitness journey and note how you are feeling along with body measurements or weight. Go ahead and take the measurements you want before you start so you can see what has changed throughout your journey. Taking

pictures of yourself before starting and at the end is another way to see a difference in how your body has changed.

The 28 Day Challenge

In this book, I have compiled several wall pilates workouts aimed at challenging you for 4 weeks. It consists of six active days of wall pilates and one rest and recovery day per week before continuing the next week of exercises. I will lay out the list of exercises and repetitions before going into the directions on how to do each exercise each day. Remember that depending on your fitness level and preferences you can adjust the repetitions, sets, or exercises to fit you. If any exercise causes discomfort you may modify or skip it. Let's get this fitness journey started!

Day 1 - Laying the Foundations

- Wall Roll-Down: 5 repetitions
- Wall Squats: 3 sets of 10 repetitions
- Wall Bridge: 3 sets of 8 repetitions
- Wall Plank: Hold for 30 seconds
- Wall Leg Lifts: 2 sets of 10 repetitions on each side

Wall Roll-Down: Stand with your back against the wall, feet about 5 inches from the wall, and hip-width apart. Slowly roll down through your spine, feeling each vertebra pull away from the wall until your head, shoulders, and spine are parallel to the floor. Hold for 3 seconds. Then roll back up to standing feeling each vertebra against the wall again. Repeat this 5 times.

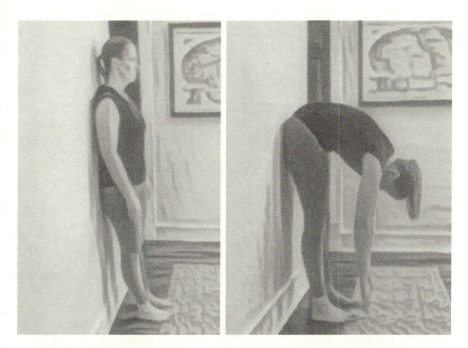

Wall Squats: Stand with your back against the wall and feet hip-width apart. Feet a little out from the wall. Slide your body down into a squat position. Keep your knees from going in front of your toes align them with your ankles and keep your back flat against the wall. Hold for 3-5 seconds, then press up through your heels to return to standing against the wall. After a few seconds continue. Repeat for 3 sets of 10 repetitions.

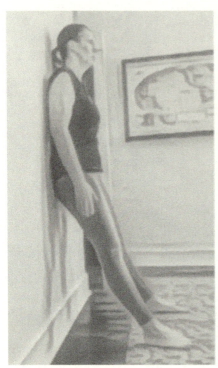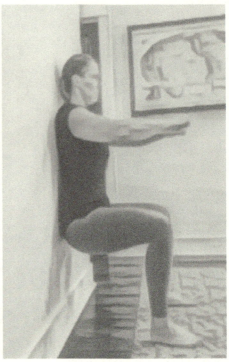

Wall Bridge: Lie on your back perpendicular to the wall. Place your feet flat on the wall with your knees bent, arms flat and supporting you. Press your feet into the wall as you lift your hips toward the ceiling, keeping your head, arms, and shoulders on the floor, and forming a bridge position. Hold for 3-5 seconds, then lower your hips back down to the floor. Repeat 3 sets of 3 repetitions.

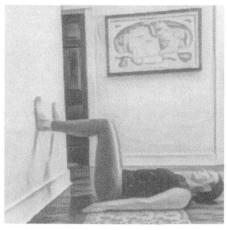
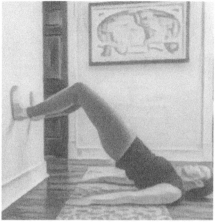

Wall Plank: Start in a push-up position with your feet against the wall and hands on the floor shoulder-width apart. Lift up your body so that it is in a straight line from head to heels. Engage your core holding your tummy in and hold for as long as you can maintain proper form or 30 seconds. Then lower yourself down and after a few seconds continue.

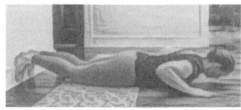
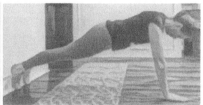

Wall Leg Lift: Stand facing the wall with your arms extended out toward the wall at shoulder height, and place your hands against the wall. Take a step back and slide your hands down to keep them at shoulder level. Engage your core by holding in your tummy and lift one leg off the ground keeping it straight behind you. Raise your leg as high as you can keeping your hips facing forward. Repeat this for 2 sets of 10 repetitions and then repeat 2 sets of 10 repetitions on the other leg.

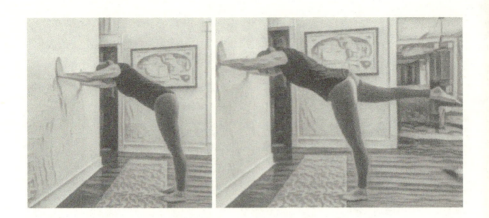

Day 2 - Focus on the Core

- Wall Roll-Down: 5 repetitions
- Wall Sit with Leg Lift: 3 sets of 8 repetitions each side
- Wall Pike: 3 sets of 8 repetitions
- Wall Side Plank: Hold for 30 seconds each side
- Wall Crunches: 2 sets of 15 repetitions

Wall Roll-Down: Stand with your back against the wall, feet about 5 inches from the wall, and hip-width apart. Slowly roll down through your spine, feeling each vertebra pull away from the wall until your head, shoulders, and spine are parallel to the floor. Hold for 3 seconds. Then roll back up to standing feeling each vertebra against the wall again. Repeat this 5 times.

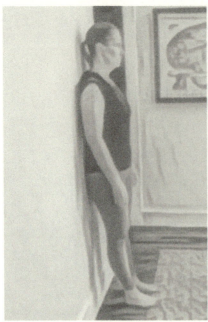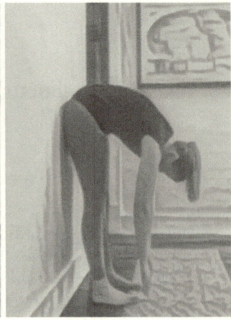

Wall Sit with Leg Lift: Stand with your back against a wall and your feet hip-width apart and away from the wall. Slide your back down the wall until your thighs are parallel to the floor, forming a seated position. Keep your knees aligned with your ankles and your back flat against the wall. Engage your core press your back against the wall and lift one leg up off the floor, keeping it straight. Hold the lifted leg for a few seconds, then lower it back down. Repeat 3 sets of 8 repetitions on each leg.

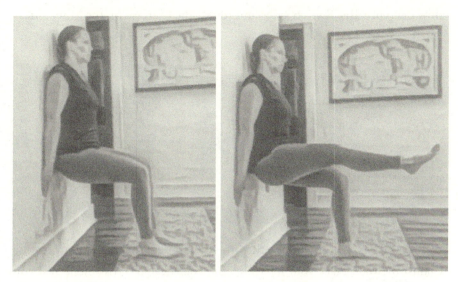

Wall Pike: Start in a plank position facing away from the wall, with your hands on the floor directly under your shoulders and your feet resting against the wall. Engage your core, lift your hips towards the ceiling, and pull your feet away from the wall coming into a pike position with your body forming an inverted "V" shape. Hold for a moment, then lower back to the starting position. Repeat for 3 sets of 8 repetitions.

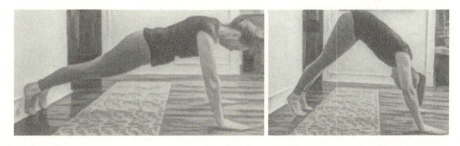

Wall Side Plank: Lie on your side with your feet against the wall and your legs extended. Place your elbow directly beneath your shoulder and prop yourself up into a side plank position. Keep your body in a straight line from head to heels, engaging your core muscles. Hold the side plank position for 30 seconds, or longer if you can maintain proper form, remembering to take slow deep breaths. Switch sides and repeat the exercise on the other side.

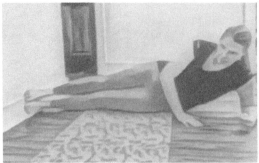 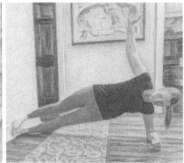

Wall Crunches: Lie on your back with your legs extended and your feet flat against the wall. Place your hands behind your head or cross them over your chest. Engage your core muscles and lift your shoulder blades off the floor, bringing your chest towards your knees. Exhale as you crunch up, inhale as you lower back down. Avoid pulling on your neck or using momentum to lift your upper body. Repeat 2 sets of 15 repetitions.

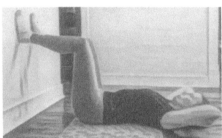 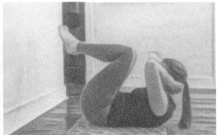

Day 3 - Lower Body

- Wall Roll-Down: 5 repetitions
- Wall Sit: Hold for 1 minute
- Wall Lunge: 3 sets of 10 repetitions each leg
- Wall Calf Raises: 3 sets of 15 repetitions
- Wall Leg Circles: 2 sets of 10 repetitions each leg (5 rotations each direction)

Wall Roll-Down: Stand with your back against the wall, feet about 5 inches from the wall, and hip-width apart. Slowly roll down through your spine, feeling each vertebra pull away from the wall until your head, shoulders, and spine are parallel to the floor. Hold for 3 seconds. Then roll back up to standing feeling each vertebra against the wall again. Repeat this 5 times.

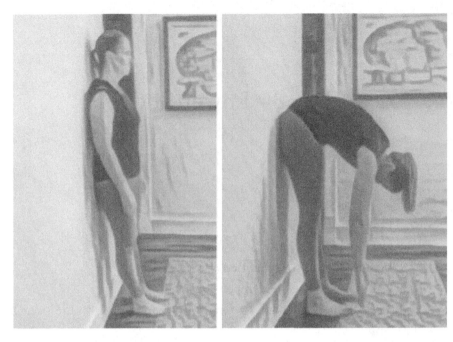

Wall Sit: Stand with your back against a wall and your feet hip-width apart, feet away from the wall. Slide your back down the wall until your thighs are parallel to the floor, forming a seated position. Keep your knees aligned with your ankles and your back flat against the wall. Hold this position for 30 seconds to 1 minute, or as long as you can maintain proper form. Focus on keeping your core engaged and your weight distributed evenly through your heels. To increase intensity, hold weight in your hands or place a resistance band around your thighs.

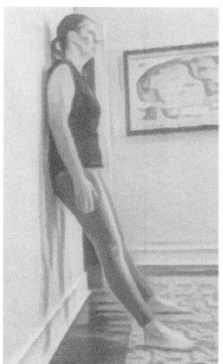 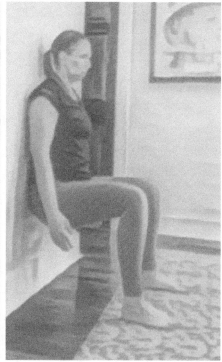

Wall Lunge: Stand about 2 feet away from a wall, facing away from it. Place one foot behind you and lean back against the wall for support. Bend your front knee to lower into a lunge position, keeping your front knee aligned with your ankle. Lower until your front thigh is parallel to the floor, making sure your back knee doesn't touch the ground. Push through your front heel to return to the starting position. Complete a set of repetitions on one leg before switching to the other leg. Repeat 3 sets of 10 repetitions on each leg.

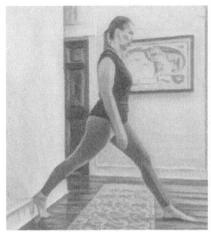 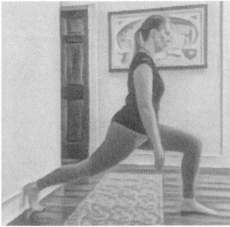

Wall Calf Raises: Stand facing a wall with your feet hip-width apart and your hands resting lightly on the wall for balance. Lift your heels off the ground as high as you can, rising onto the balls of your feet. Hold the top position for a moment, then lower your heels back down to the starting position. Make sure to control the movement throughout and avoid bouncing. Repeat 3 sets of 15 repetitions.

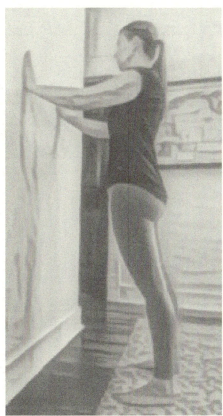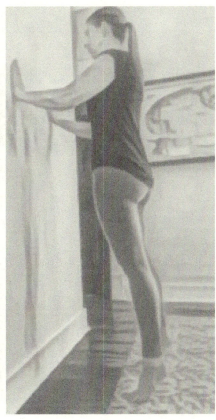

Wall Leg Circles: Lie on your back with your hips close to the wall and your feet against the wall similar to a bridge. Place your hands on the floor by your sides for support. Lift your hips off the floor, engage your core muscles, and slowly lower one leg to the side in a circular motion, keeping it straight. Continue the circle until your leg returns to the starting position. Repeat 5 times. Reverse the direction of the circle and repeat the movement. Complete a set of repetitions on one leg before switching to the other leg. Repeat 2 sets of 10 repetitions for each leg (5 each direction). Remember to breathe throughout the exercise.

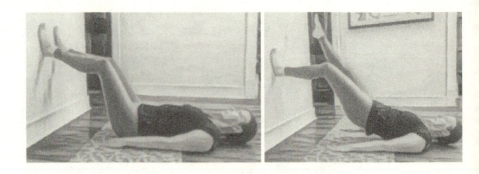

Day 4 - Upper Body

- Wall Roll-Down: 5 repetitions
- Wall Push-Ups: 3 sets of 10 repetitions
- Wall Tricep Dips: 3 sets of 10 repetitions
- Wall Shoulder Taps: 2 sets of 15 repetitions each side
- Wall Arm Circles: 2 sets of 15 repetitions forward and backward

Wall Roll-Down: Stand with your back against the wall, feet about 5 inches from the wall, and hip-width apart. Slowly roll down through your spine, feeling each vertebra pull away from the wall until your head, shoulders, and spine are parallel to the floor. Hold for 3 seconds. Then roll back up to standing feeling each vertebra against the wall again. Repeat this 5 times.

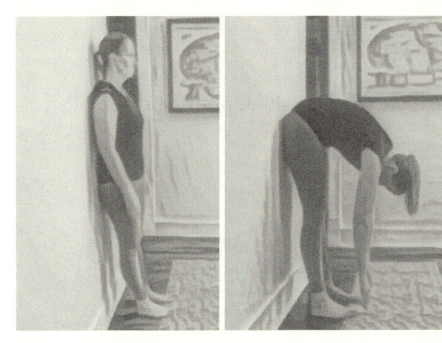

Wall Push-Ups: Stand facing a wall at arm's length, with your feet hip-width apart. Place your hands flat against the wall at shoulder height, slightly wider than shoulder width apart. Lean forward and brace your core, keeping your body in a straight line from head to heels. Bend your elbows and lower your chest towards the wall, keeping your elbows close to your body. Push through your palms to straighten your arms and return to the starting position. Repeat 3 sets of 10 repetitions. Take a step back or more to increase difficulty.

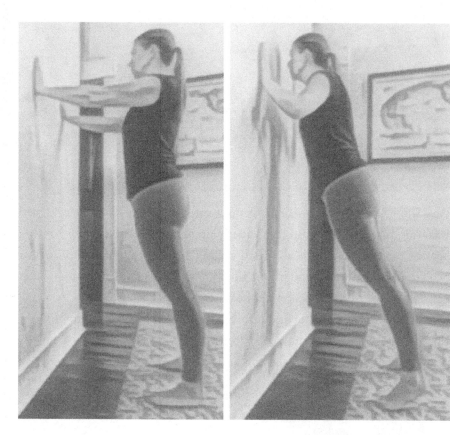

Wall Tricep Dips: Sit on the floor with your feet against the wall, knees bent. Lean back and place your hands on the floor, elbows bent, and fingers pointing towards your feet. Engage your core, press through your palms to lift your hips off the floor, straightening your arms. Lower your hips towards the floor by bending your elbows. Keep your bottom off the floor and elbows close to your body to engage triceps. Repeat 3 sets of 10 repetitions.

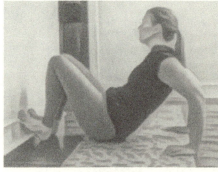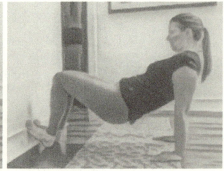

Wall Shoulder Taps: Start in a plank position facing away from the wall, with your hands on the floor directly under your shoulders and your feet resting against the wall. Brace your core to keep your body in a straight line from head to heels. Lift one hand off the floor and tap the opposite shoulder, then return it to the floor. Repeat with the other hand, alternating sides with each tap. Keep your hips stable and minimize any twisting or swaying motion. Repeat 2 sets of 15 repetitions on each shoulder.

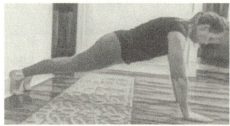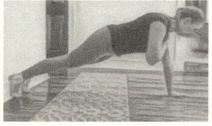

Wall Arm Circles: Stand facing the wall with your arms extended out toward the wall at shoulder height, pressing your palms flat against the wall. Begin making circular motions with your arms, moving them forward in small circles. Gradually increase the size of the circles, keeping your arms straight and shoulders relaxed. After completing forward circles, reverse the direction and perform circles in the opposite direction. Repeat 2 sets of 15 forward and backward.

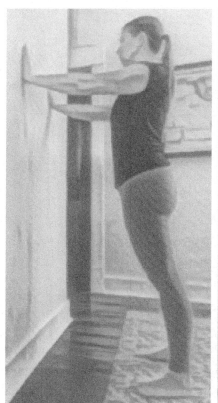 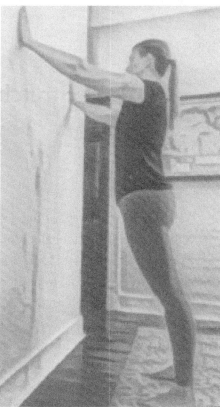

Day 5 - Stretch for Flexibility

- Wall Roll-Down: 5 repetitions
- Wall Hamstring Stretch: Hold for 30 seconds each leg
- Wall Chest Opener: Hold for 30 seconds
- Wall Figure-4 Stretch: Hold for 30 seconds each leg
- Wall Quad Stretch: Hold for 30 seconds each leg

Wall Roll-Down: Stand with your back against the wall, feet about 5 inches from the wall, and hip-width apart. Slowly roll down through your spine, feeling each vertebra pull away from the wall until your head, shoulders, and spine are parallel to the floor. Hold for 3 seconds. Then roll back up to standing feeling each vertebra against the wall again. Repeat this 5 times.

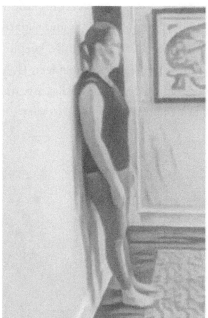 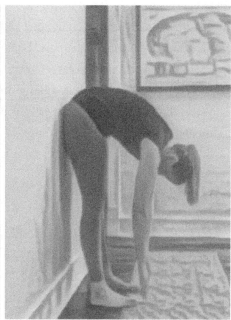

Wall Hamstring Stretch: Lie on your back with your hips close to a wall and your legs extended upward, pressing against the wall. Keep your legs straight and flex your feet towards you. Slowly slide one leg down the wall, keeping it straight, until you feel a stretch in the back of your thigh (hamstring). Hold the stretch for 30 seconds. Switch legs and repeat the stretch on the other side.

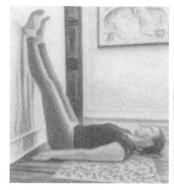 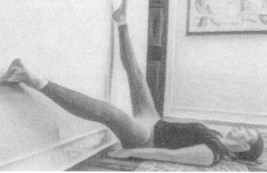

Wall Chest Opener: Stand facing away from a wall with your feet hip-width apart. Place your hands flat against the wall at shoulder height and slightly wider than shoulder width apart. Lean your body forward slightly, keeping your arms straight, until you feel a stretch in your chest and shoulders. Hold the stretch for 30 seconds, focusing on breathing deeply and relaxing into the stretch. You can adjust the height of your hands on the wall to vary the intensity of the stretch.

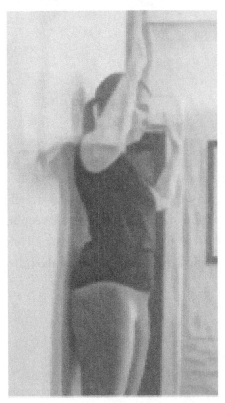
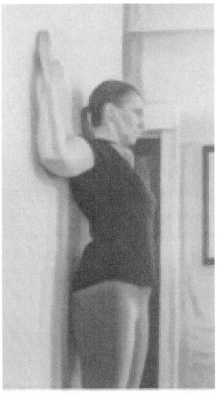

Wall Figure-4 Stretch: Lie on your back with your hips close to a wall and your legs extended up and against the wall. Cross one ankle over the opposite knee, forming a figure-4 shape with your legs. Slowly slide your foot which is still against the wall, down the wall until you feel a stretch in your outer hip and glute. Hold the stretch for 30 seconds. Switch legs and repeat the stretch on the other side.

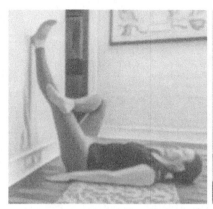 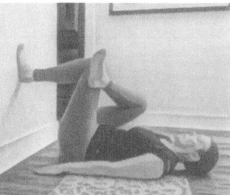

Wall Quad Stretch: Stand facing a wall and place one hand against it for balance. Bend one knee and bring your heel towards your buttocks, grasping your ankle with your free hand. Gently pull your heel towards your buttocks until you feel a stretch in the front of your thigh (quadriceps). Keep your knees close together and your torso upright. Hold the stretch for 30 seconds. Switch legs and repeat the stretch on the other side.

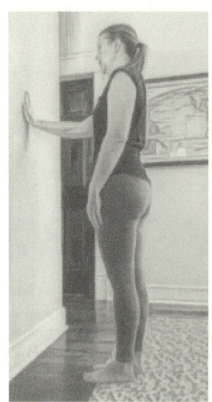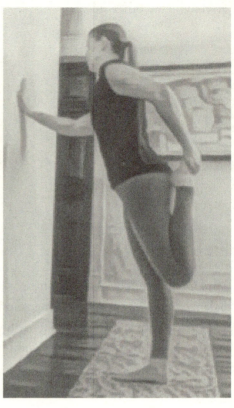

Day 6 - Flow

- Wall Roll-Down: 5 repetitions
- Wall Plank to Downward Dog: 3 sets of 8 repetitions
- Wall Squat to Overhead Reach: 3 sets of 10 repetitions
- Wall Bridge with Leg Lift: 3 sets of 8 repetitions each leg
- Wall Side Plank with Rotation: 2 sets of 10 repetitions each side

Wall Roll-Down: Stand with your back against the wall, feet about 5 inches from the wall, and hip-width apart. Slowly roll down through your spine, feeling each vertebra pull away from the wall until your head, shoulders, and spine are parallel to the floor. Hold for 3 seconds. Then roll back up to standing feeling each vertebra against the wall again. Repeat this 5 times.

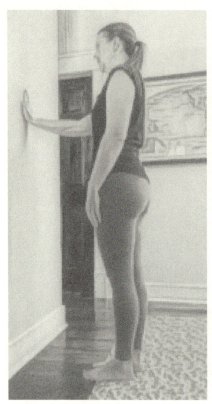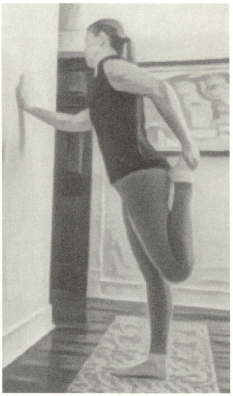

Wall Plank to Downward Dog: Start in a plank position facing away from the wall, with your hands on the floor directly under your shoulders and your feet resting against the wall. Keep your body in a straight line from head to heels. Press through your palms and push your hips up towards the ceiling, shifting into a downward dog position. Your body should form an inverted "V" shape, with your arms and back straight and your heels pressing towards the floor. Hold the downward dog position for a few seconds, then return to the plank position. Make sure to focus on smooth and controlled movements. Repeat 3 sets of 8 repetitions.

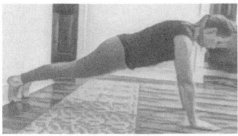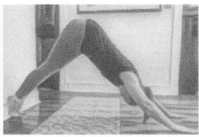

Wall Squat to Overhead Reach: Stand with your back against a wall and your feet hip-width apart, a few feet away from the wall. Lower into a squat position, sliding your back down the wall until your thighs are parallel to the floor and your knees are at a 90-degree angle. Keep your knees aligned with your ankles and your back flat against the wall. From the squat position, push through your heels to stand up straight while simultaneously reaching your arms overhead. Extend your arms fully towards the ceiling, keeping them straight. Lower your arms back down to shoulder height as you return to the squat position. Try focusing on maintaining good form throughout the movement. Repeat for 3 sets of 10 repetitions.

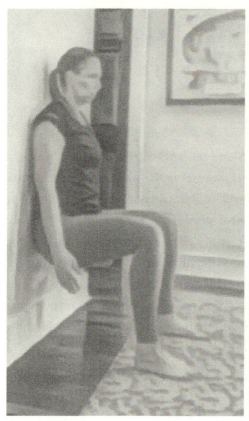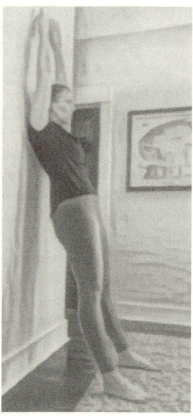

Wall Bridge with Leg Lift: Lie on your back with your feet flat on the floor and your knees bent, close to a wall. Press your feet into the wall and lift your hips off the floor, coming into a bridge position. Keep your shoulders and upper back on the floor and engage your core and glutes to support your body. From the bridge position, lift one leg off the wall and extend it straight towards the ceiling. Hold the lifted leg for a few seconds, then lower it back down. Continue on the same leg. Repeat for 3 sets of 8 repetitions for each leg.

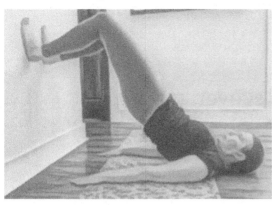 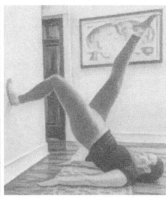

Wall Side Plank with Rotation: Start in a side plank position with your forearm on the floor and your feet stacked. Lift your hips off the floor, keeping your body in a straight line from head to heels. Extend your opposite arm towards the ceiling. From the side plank position, rotate your torso reaching your top arm underneath your body. Rotate back to the starting side plank position, extending your arm towards the ceiling. Focus on controlled movements and maintaining stability in the plank position. Repeat for 2 sets of 10 repetitions on each side.

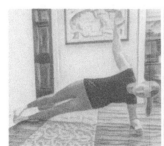 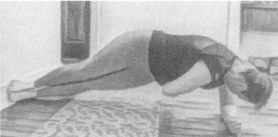

Day 7 - Recover and Reflect

- Stretching: Spend 10-15 minutes stretching areas of tension or tightness.
- Reflect: Take a moment to reflect on your progress. Write down or mentally note improvements in strength and flexibility, or overall feelings of well-being.
- Rest: Allow your body to recharge.

Day 8 - Strengthen Your Core

- Wall Roll-Down: 5 repetitions
- Wall Plank with Leg Lift: 3 sets of 8 repetitions each side
- Wall Pike: 3 sets of 8 repetitions
- Wall side plank: Hold for 30 seconds each side
- Wall Crunches: 2 sets of 15 repetitions

Wall Roll-Down: Stand with your back against the wall, feet about 5 inches from the wall, and hip-width apart. Slowly roll down through your spine, feeling each vertebra pull away from the wall until your head, shoulders, and spine are parallel to the floor. Hold for 3 seconds. Then roll back up to standing feeling each vertebra against the wall again. Repeat this 5 times.

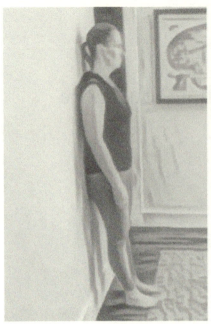
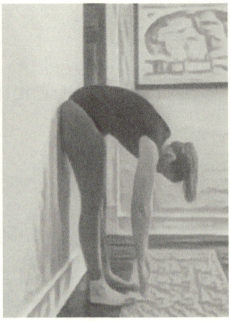

Wall Plank with Leg Lift: Start in a plank position facing away from the wall. Place your hands on the floor directly under your shoulders and your feet resting against the wall. Walk your feet up the wall a little until your body is in a straight line, similar to a traditional plank position. Engage your core and lift one leg up off the wall, keeping it straight. Hold the lifted leg for a few seconds, then lower it back down. Repeat 3 sets of 8 repetitions on each leg. Keep your feet dry for stability.

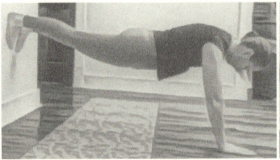
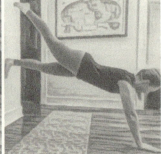

Wall Pike: Start in a plank position facing away from the wall, with your hands on the floor directly under your shoulders and your feet resting against the wall. Engage your core, lift your hips towards the ceiling, and pull your feet away from the wall coming into a pike position with your body forming an inverted "V" shape. Hold for a moment, then lower back to the starting position. Repeat for 3 sets of 8 repetitions.

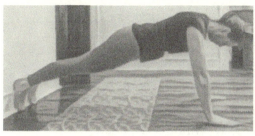 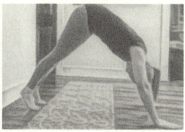

Wall Crunches: Lie on your back with your legs extended and your feet flat against the wall. Place your hands behind your head or cross them over your chest. Engage your core muscles and lift your shoulder blades off the floor, bringing your chest towards your knees. Exhale as you crunch up, inhale as you lower back down. Avoid pulling on your neck or using momentum to lift your upper body. Repeat 2 sets of 15 repetitions.

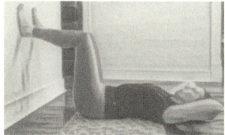 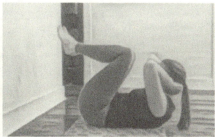

Day 9 - Strengthen Upper Body

- Wall Roll-Down: 5 repetitions
- Wall Push-Ups: 3 sets of 10 repetitions
- Wall Tricep Dips: 3 sets of 10 repetitions
- Wall Shoulder Taps: 2 sets of 15 repetitions each side
- Wall Arm Circles: 2 sets of 15 repetitions forward and backward

Wall Roll-Down: Stand with your back against the wall, feet about 5 inches from the wall, and hip-width apart. Slowly roll down through your spine, feeling each vertebra pull away from the wall until your head, shoulders, and spine are parallel to the floor. Hold for 3 seconds. Then roll back up to standing feeling each vertebra against the wall again. Repeat this 5 times.

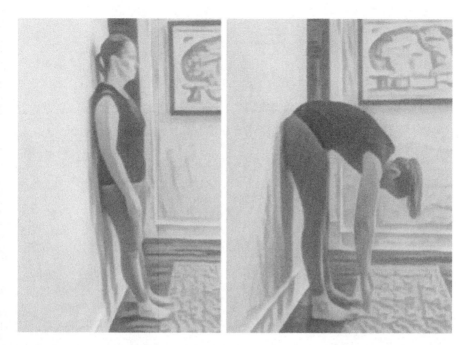

Wall Push-Ups: Stand facing a wall at arm's length, with your feet hip-width apart. Place your hands flat against the wall at shoulder height, slightly wider than shoulder width apart. Lean forward and brace your core, keeping your body in a straight line from head to heels. Bend your elbows and lower your chest towards the wall, keeping your elbows close to your body. Push through your palms to straighten your arms and return to the starting position. Repeat 3 sets of 10 repetitions. Take a step back or more to increase difficulty.

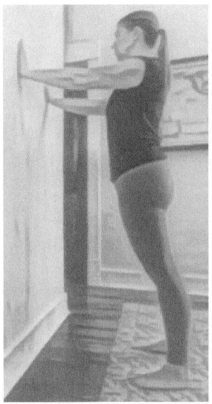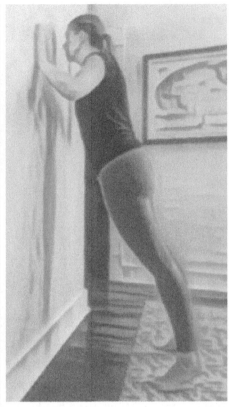

Wall Tricep Dips: Sit on the floor with your back against the wall, knees bent, and feet flat on the floor. Place your hands on the floor beside your hips, fingers pointing towards your feet. Press through your palms to lift your hips off the floor, straightening your arms. You can step your feet out a little bit and raise your core a little, coming to a reverse table-top position. Lower your hips towards the floor by bending your elbows, keeping them close to your body. Don't worry about staying against the wall. Push through your palms to straighten your arms and return to the starting position. Repeat 3 sets of 10 repetitions.

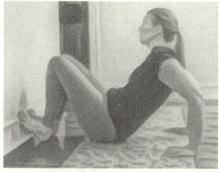 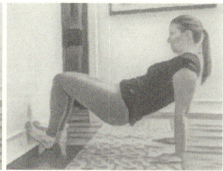

Wall Shoulder Taps: Start in a plank position facing away from the wall, with your hands on the floor directly under your shoulders and your feet resting against the wall. Brace your core to keep your body in a straight line from head to heels. Lift one hand off the floor and tap the opposite shoulder, then return it to the floor. Repeat with the other hand, alternating sides with each tap. Keep your hips stable and minimize any twisting or swaying motion. Repeat 2 sets of 15 repetitions on each shoulder.

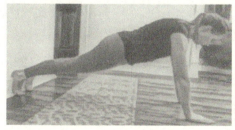 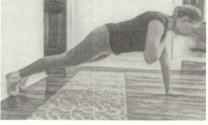

Wall Arm Circles: Stand facing the wall with your arms extended out toward the wall at shoulder height, pressing your palms flat against the wall. Begin making circular motions with your arms, moving them forward in small circles. Gradually increase the size of the circles, keeping your arms straight and shoulders relaxed. After completing forward circles, reverse the direction and perform circles in the opposite direction. Repeat 2 sets of 15 forward and backward.

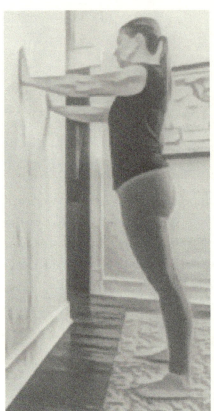 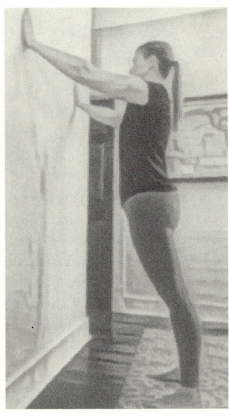

Day 10 - Focus on Lower Body

- Wall Roll-Down: 5 repetitions
- Wall Squats: 3 sets of 12 repetitions
- Wall Lunges: 3 sets of 10 repetitions each leg
- Wall Calf Raises: 3 sets of 15 repetitions
- Wall Bridge: Hold for 30 seconds

Wall Roll-Down: Stand with your back against the wall, feet about 5 inches from the wall, and hip-width apart. Slowly roll down through your spine, feeling each vertebra pull away from the wall until your head, shoulders, and spine are parallel to the floor. Hold for 3 seconds. Then roll back up to standing feeling each vertebra against the wall again. Repeat this 5 times.

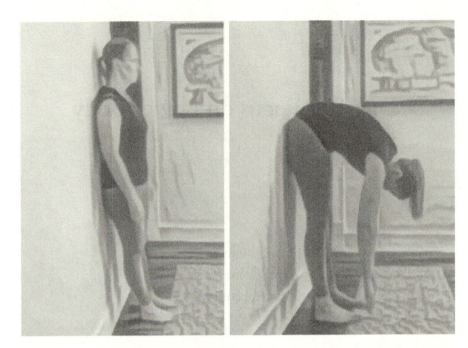

Wall Squats: Stand with your back against the wall and feet hip-width apart. Feet a little out from the wall. Slide your body down into a squat position. Keep your knees from going in front of your toes align them with your ankles and keep your back flat against the wall. Hold for 3-5 seconds, then press up through your heels to return to standing against the wall. After a few seconds continue. Repeat for 3 sets of 12 repetitions.

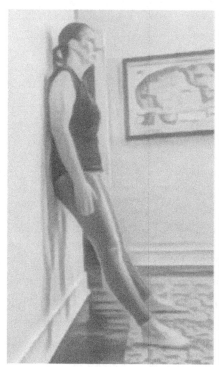 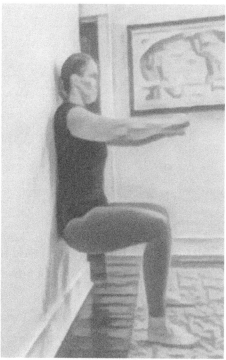

Wall Lunge: Stand about 2 feet away from a wall, facing away from it. Place one foot behind you and lean back against the wall for support. Bend your front knee to lower into a lunge position, keeping your front knee aligned with your ankle. Lower until your front thigh is parallel to the floor, making sure your back knee doesn't touch the ground. Push through your front heel to return to the starting position. Complete a set of repetitions on one leg before switching to the other leg. Repeat 3 sets of 10 repetitions on each leg.

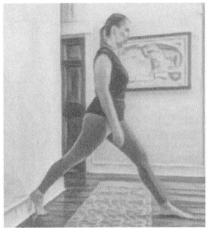 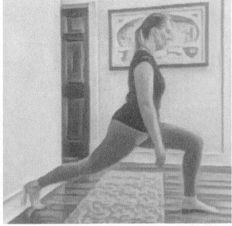

Wall Calf Raise Instructions: Stand facing a wall with your feet hip-width apart and your hands resting lightly on the wall for balance. Lift your heels off the ground as high as you can, rising onto the balls of your feet. Hold the top position for a moment, then lower your heels back down to the starting position. Make sure to control the movement throughout and avoid bouncing. Repeat 3 sets of 15 repetitions.

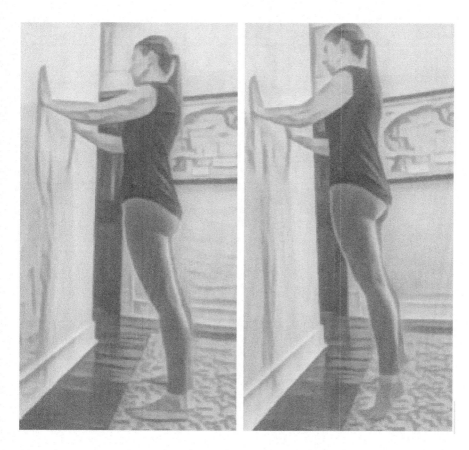

Wall Bridge: Lie on your back perpendicular to the wall. Place your feet flat on the wall with your knees bent, arms flat and supporting you. Press your feet into the wall as you lift your hips toward the ceiling, keeping your head, arms, and shoulders on the floor, and forming a bridge position. Hold for 30 seconds, then lower your hips back down to the floor.

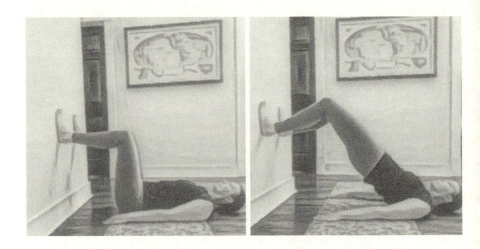

Day 11 - Balance and Stability

- Wall Roll-Down: 5 repetitions
- Wall Single-Leg Squats: 3 sets of 8 repetitions each leg
- Wall Plank with Knee Tucks: 3 sets of 8 repetitions
- Wall Single-Leg Balance: 2 sets of 30 seconds each leg
- Wall Leg Swings: 2 sets of 10 repetitions each leg

Wall Roll-Down: Stand with your back against the wall, feet about 5 inches from the wall, and hip-width apart. Slowly roll down through your spine, feeling each vertebra pull away from the wall until your head, shoulders, and spine are parallel to the floor. Hold for 3 seconds. Then roll back up to standing feeling each vertebra against the wall again. Repeat this 5 times.

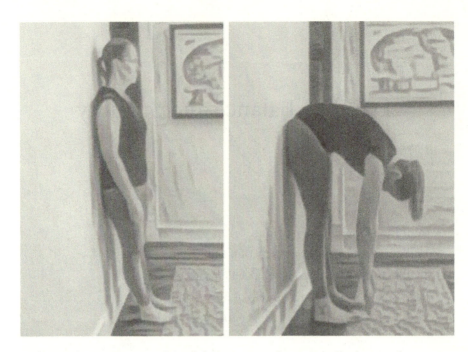

Wall Single-Leg Squats: Stand facing away from a wall, about a foot or so away, with your feet hip-width apart, and lean against the wall. Extend one leg straight out in front of you, hovering it off the ground. Place your hands on the wall, on your hips or extend them in front of you for balance. Slowly lower your body into a squat position by bending your standing leg, keeping your back straight and chest up. Lower down as far as you can while maintaining balance and control. Push through your heel to return to the starting position. Repeat 3 sets of 8 repetitions on each leg.

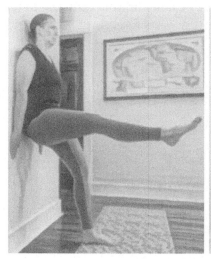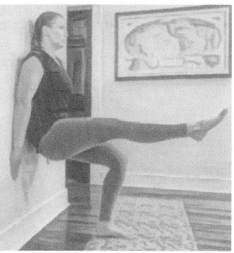

Wall Plank with Knee Tucks: Start in a plank position facing away from a wall, with your hands on the floor directly under your shoulders and your feet resting against the wall. Keep your body in a straight line from head to heels, engaging your core and glutes. Slowly bring one knee towards your chest, keeping your hips level and your back flat. Return the leg to the starting position and repeat with the other leg. Repeat 3 sets of 8 repetitions on each leg, alternating sides.

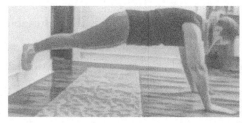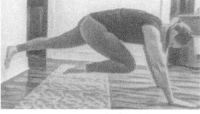

Wall Single-Leg Balance: Stand facing a wall and place one hand lightly on the wall for balance. Lift one foot off the ground and balance on the other foot. Keep your standing leg slightly bent and your core engaged to help maintain balance. Hold the position for 20-30 seconds, focusing on keeping your body stable. Switch legs and repeat the balance on the other leg. To increase difficulty, try closing your eyes or extending your arms out to the sides for balance. Do 2 sets for 30 seconds each leg.

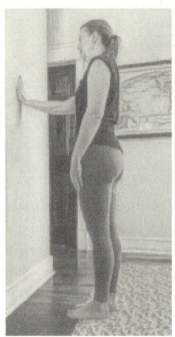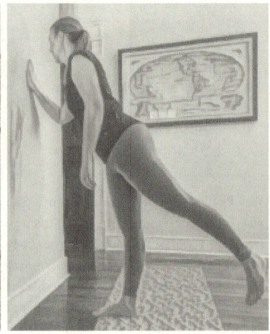

Wall Leg Swings: Stand sideways to a wall and place one hand lightly on the wall for support. Swing your outside leg forward and backward in a controlled motion, keeping it straight. Swing your leg as high as comfortable, but avoid forcing it beyond your range of motion. Focus on keeping your torso stable and engaging your core muscles. Perform 10 swings on one leg, then switch sides and repeat with the other leg. Do 2 sets of 10 repetitions on each leg.

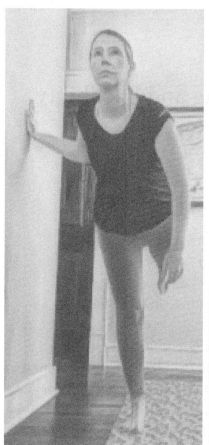 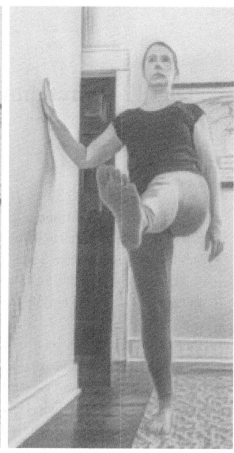

Day 12 - Stretching and Flexibility

- Wall Roll-Down: 5 repetitions
- Wall Hamstring Stretch: Hold for 30 seconds each leg
- Wall Chest Opener Stretch: Hold for 30 seconds
- Wall Quadriceps Stretch: Hold for 30 seconds each leg
- Wall Spinal Twist Stretch: Hold for 30 seconds each side

Wall Roll-Down: Stand with your back against the wall, feet about 5 inches from the wall, and hip-width apart. Slowly roll down through your spine, feeling each vertebra pull away from the wall until your head, shoulders, and spine are parallel to the floor. Hold for 3 seconds. Then roll back up to standing feeling each vertebra against the wall again. Repeat this 5 times.

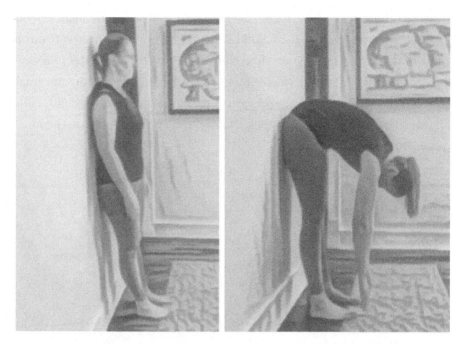

Wall Hamstring Stretch: Lie on your back with your hips close to a wall and your legs extended upward, pressing against the wall. Keep your legs straight and flex your feet towards you. Slowly slide one leg down the wall, keeping it straight, until you feel a stretch in the back of your thigh (hamstring). Hold the stretch for 30 seconds. Switch legs and repeat the stretch on the other side.

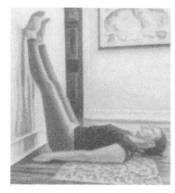
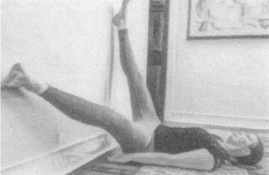

Wall Quad Stretch: Stand facing away from a wall with one hand resting lightly on the wall for balance. Bend one knee and bring your heel towards your buttocks, grasping your ankle with your free hand. Gently pull your heel towards your buttocks until you feel a stretch in the front of your thigh (quadriceps). Keep your knees close together and your torso upright. Hold the stretch for 30 seconds. Switch legs and repeat the stretch on the other side.

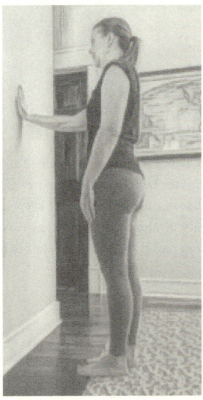
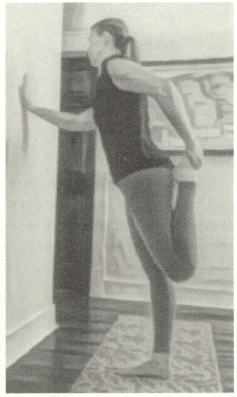

Wall Spinal Twist Stretch: Sit on the floor with your right side close to a wall. Lie on your back and swing your legs up against the wall, so your body forms an "L" shape, with your hips close to the wall and your legs extended vertically. Extend your arms out to the sides in a T-position, palms facing up. Lower both legs to the right side, allowing them to rest against the wall. Turn your head to the left and gaze in the opposite direction of your legs. Feel the stretch along your spine and through your chest and shoulders. Hold the stretch for 30 seconds, then return to the starting position. Repeat on the other side by lowering your legs to the left and turning your head to the right.

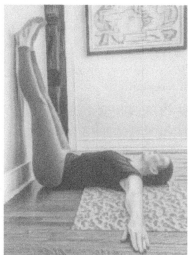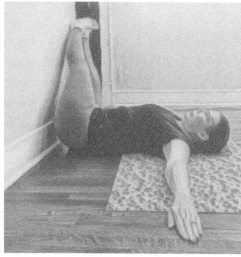

Day 13 - Flow

- Wall Roll-Down: 5 repetitions
- Wall Plank to Downward Dog: 3 sets of 8 repetitions
- Wall Squat to Overhead Reach: 3 sets of 10 repetitions
- Wall Bridge with Leg Lift: 3 sets of 8 repetitions each leg
- Wall Side Plank with Rotation: 2 sets of 10 repetitions each side

Wall Roll-Down: Stand with your back against the wall, feet about 5 inches from the wall and hip-width apart. Slowly roll down through your spine, feeling each vertebra pull away from the wall until your head, shoulders, and spine are parallel to the floor. Hold for 3 seconds. Then roll back up to standing feeling each vertebra against the wall again. Repeat this 5 times.

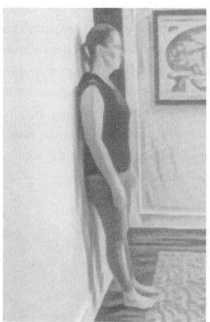 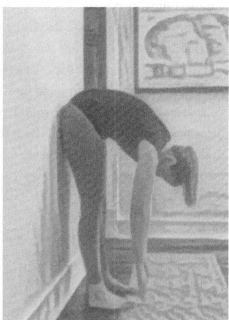

Wall Plank to Downward Dog: Start in a plank position facing away from the wall, with your hands shoulder-width apart and your feet hip-width apart. Keep your body in a straight line from head to heels. Press through your palms and push your hips up towards the ceiling, shifting into a downward dog position. Your body should form an inverted "V" shape, with your arms and back straight and your heels pressing towards the floor. Hold the downward dog position for a few seconds, then return to the plank position. Make sure to focus on smooth and controlled movements. Repeat 3 sets of 8 repetitions.

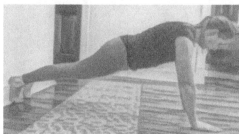 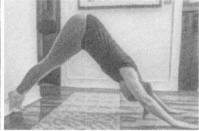

Wall Squat to Overhead Reach: Stand with your back against a wall and your feet hip-width apart, a few feet away from the wall. Lower into a squat position, sliding your back down the wall until your thighs are parallel to the floor and your knees are at a 90-degree angle. Keep your knees aligned with your ankles and your back flat against the wall. From the squat position, push through your heels to stand up straight while simultaneously reaching your arms overhead. Extend your arms fully towards the ceiling, keeping them straight. Lower your arms back down to shoulder height as you return to the squat position. Try focusing on maintaining good form throughout the movement. Repeat for 3 sets of 10 repetitions.

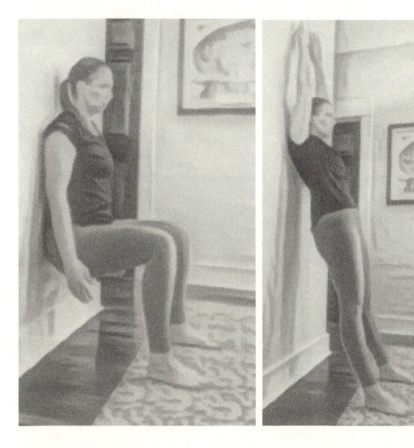

Wall Bridge with Leg Lift: Lie on your back with your feet flat on the floor and your knees bent, close to a wall. Press your feet into the wall and lift your hips off the floor, coming into a bridge position. Keep your shoulders and upper back on the floor and engage your core and glutes to support your body. From the bridge position, lift one leg off the wall and extend it straight towards the ceiling. Hold the lifted leg for a few seconds, then lower it back down. Continue on the same leg. Repeat for 3 sets of 8 repetitions for each leg.

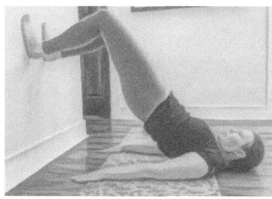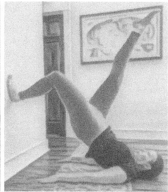

Wall Side Plank with Rotation: Start in a side plank position facing the wall, with your forearm on the floor and your feet stacked. Lift your hips off the floor, keeping your body in a straight line from head to heels. Extend your opposite arm towards the ceiling. From the side plank position, rotate your torso, reaching your top arm underneath your body. Rotate back to the starting side plank position, extending your arm towards the ceiling. Focus on controlled movements and maintaining stability in the plank position. Repeat for 2 sets of 10 repetitions on each side.

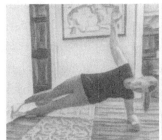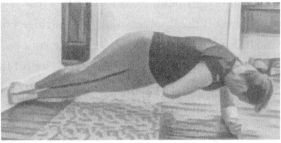

Day 14 - Recover and Rest

- Stretching: Spend 10-15 minutes stretching areas of tension or tightness.
- Reflect: Take a moment to reflect on your progress. Write down or mentally note improvements in strength and flexibility, or overall feelings of well-being.
- Rest: Allow your body to recharge.

Day 15 - Core Strength

- Wall Roll-Down to Twist: 5 repetitions each side
- Wall Plank with Alternating Leg Lifts: 3 sets of 8 repetitions each side
- Wall Pike to Knee Tucks: 3 sets of 8 repetitions
- Wall Side Plank with Hip Dips: 3 sets of 8 repetitions each side
- Wall Crunches with Rotation: 2 sets of 15 repetitions each side

Wall Roll-Down to Twist: Start by standing tall with your back against the wall, feet hip-width apart. Engage your core and slowly begin to roll down towards the floor, one vertebra at a time, until your hands can touch the ground. Once your hands are on the ground, walk them out in front of you until you are in a plank position with your hands directly under your shoulders. Rotate your body to one side, lifting one arm towards the ceiling while keeping your hips square. Hold the twist for a moment, then return to plank position. Repeat the twist on the opposite side. Walk your hands back towards your feet and slowly roll back up to standing, one vertebra at a time. Do 5 repetitions on each side.

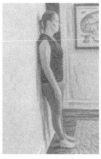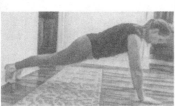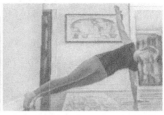

Wall Plank with Alternating Leg Lifts: Start in a plank position facing away from the wall, with your hands on the floor directly under your shoulders and your feet resting against the wall. Engage your core and lift one foot off the wall, bringing your knee towards your chest. Hold for a moment, then return your foot to the wall. Repeat the leg lift on the opposite side. Continue alternating legs for 3 sets of 8 repetitions on each side.

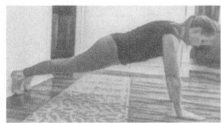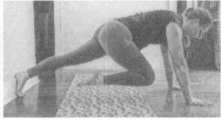

Wall Pike to Knee Tucks: Start in a plank position facing away from the wall, with your hands on the floor directly under your shoulders and your feet resting against the wall. Engage your core, lift your hips towards the ceiling, and pull your feet away from the wall coming into a pike position with your body forming an inverted "V". Hold for a moment, then bend your knees and pull them towards your chest, coming into a knee tuck position. Extend your legs back out to the pike position. Repeat for 3 sets of 8 repetitions.

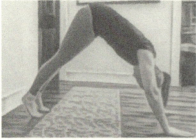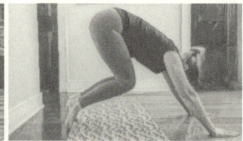

Wall Side Plank with Hip Dips: Start in a side plank position facing the wall, with your forearm on the floor and your feet stacked. Lift your hips off the floor, keeping your body in a straight line from head to heels. Lower your hips towards the floor, then lift them back up towards the ceiling. Repeat for 3 sets of 8 repetitions on each side.

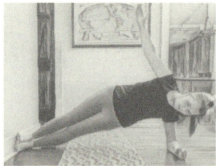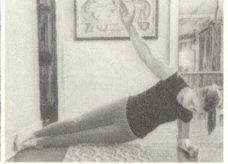

Wall Crunches with Rotation: Lie on your back with your hips close to the wall and your knees bent, feet flat on the floor. Place your hands lightly behind your head, elbows pointing out to the sides. Engage your core and lift your shoulder blades off the floor, bringing your chest towards your knees. As you crunch up, rotate your torso to one side, bringing your elbow towards the opposite knee. Return to the center and lower back down. Repeat the crunch, this time rotating to the opposite side. Continue alternating sides for 2 sets of 15 repetitions each side.

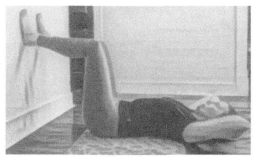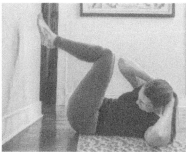

Day 16 - Upper Body

- Wall Roll-Down: 5 repetitions
- Wall Push-Ups with Leg Extension: 3 sets of 10 repetitions
- Wall Tricep Press: 3 sets of 10 repetitions
- Wall Shoulder Press: 3 sets of 10 repetitions
- Wall Arm Circles: 2 sets of 20 repetitions forward and backward

Wall Roll-Down: Stand with your back against the wall, feet about 5 inches from the wall and hip-width apart. Slowly roll down through your spine, feeling each vertebra pull away from the wall until your head, shoulders and spine are parallel to the floor. Hold for 3 seconds. Then roll back up to standing feeling each vertebra against the wall again. Repeat this 5 times.

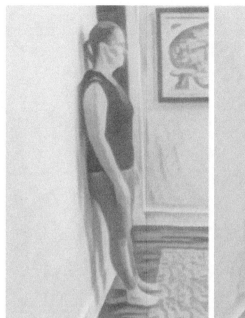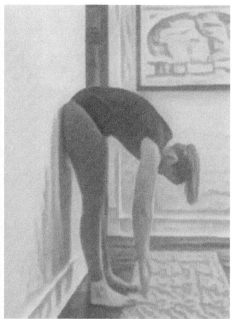

Wall Push-Ups with Leg Extension: Stand facing a wall with your arms extended at shoulder height, palms flat against the wall and slightly wider than shoulder-width apart. Step your feet back a few feet from the wall, keeping them hip-width apart. Engage your core and maintain a straight line from your head to your heels. Bend your elbows to lower your chest towards the wall, keeping your body in a straight line. As you push back up, simultaneously lift one leg off the ground and extend it straight behind you. Lower your leg back down as you bend your elbows to perform another push-up. Alternate legs with each repetition. Repeat 3 sets of 10 repetitions on each leg.

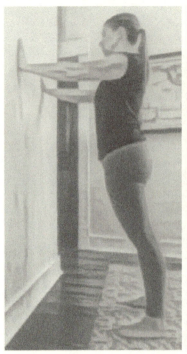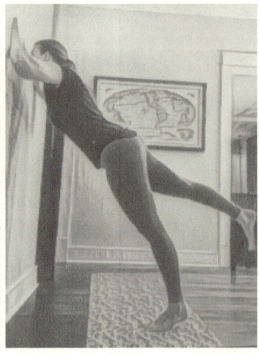

Wall Tricep Press: Stand facing a wall and place your palms flat against the wall at shoulder height and slightly closer in than shoulder width apart. Step your feet back a few feet from the wall, keeping them hip-width apart. Lean your body forward slightly, keeping your arms straight. Bend your elbows to lower your chest towards the wall, keeping your elbows close to your body. Press through your palms to straighten your arms and return to the starting position. Focus on squeezing your triceps at the top of the movement. Repeat for 3 sets of 10 repetitions.

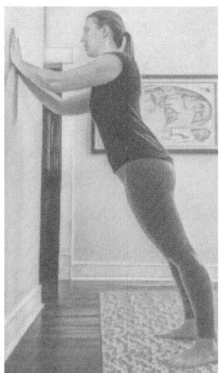 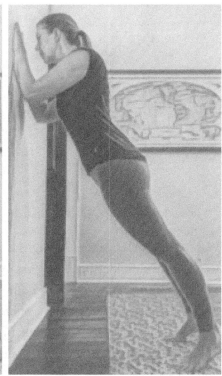

Wall Shoulder Press: Stand facing a wall with your feet hip-width apart.
Extend your arms straight in front of you at shoulder height, palms facing the wall. Lean forward slightly and brace your core. Bend your elbows to lower your chest towards the wall, keeping your upper arms parallel to the floor. Press through your palms to push yourself away from the wall, extending your arms fully overhead. Lower your arms back down to shoulder height to complete one repetition. Repeat for 3 sets of 10 repetitions. Remember to maintain proper form.

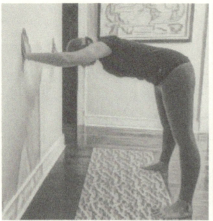 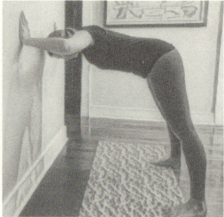

Wall Arm Circles: Stand facing the wall with your arms extended out to the sides at shoulder height. Press your palms flat against the wall. Begin making circular motions with your arms, moving them forward in small circles. Gradually increase the size of the circles, keeping your arms straight and shoulders relaxed. After completing forward circles, reverse the direction and perform circles in the opposite direction. Repeat 2 sets of 20 forward and backward.

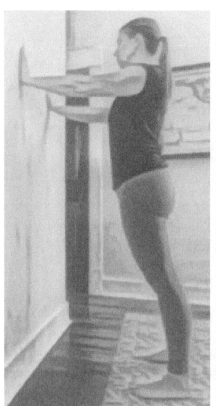 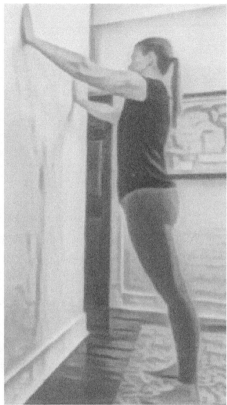

Day 17 - Lower Body

- Wall Roll-Down to Forward Lunge: 5 repetitions each leg
- Wall Squat Pulses: 3 sets of 15 repetitions
- Wall Side Leg Raises: 3 sets of 12 repetitions each leg
- Wall Calf Raises with Hold: 3 sets of 15 repetitions
- Wall Bridge with Leg Extension: 2 sets of 10 repetitions each leg

Wall Roll-Down to Forward Lunge: Stand with your back against the wall, feet about 5 inches from the wall and hip-width apart. Slowly roll down through your spine, feeling each vertebra pull away from the wall until your head, shoulders and spine are parallel to the floor. Walk your hands forward until you are in a plank position with your hands directly under your shoulders. Step one foot forward between your hands into a lunge position. Lower your back knee towards the ground until both knees are bent at 90-degree angles. Push through your front heel to return to standing, then step your foot back to plank position. Walk your hands back towards your feet and slowly roll back up to standing against the wall, one vertebra at a time. Repeat the movement, alternating legs for each lunge for 5 repetitions on each leg.

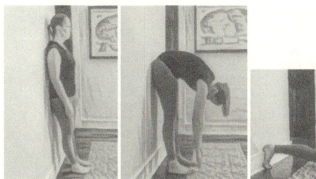
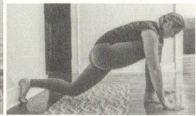

Wall Squat Pulses: Stand with your back against a wall and your feet hip-width apart, a few feet away from the wall. Lower into a squat position by bending your knees and sliding your back down the wall until your thighs are parallel to the floor and your knees are at a 90-degree angle. Hold this position and pulse up and down slightly, moving only a few inches. Keep your back flat against the wall and your knees aligned with your ankles. Do 3 sets of 15 repetitions.

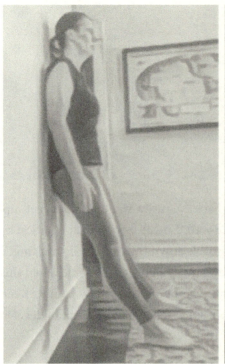 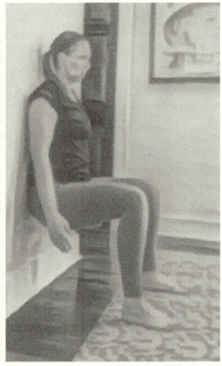

Wall Side Leg Raises: Stand sideways to a wall with one hand lightly resting on the wall for balance. Lift your outside leg out to the side as high as you can, keeping it straight. Lower your leg back down to the starting position with control. Repeat for 3 sets of 12 repetitions on each leg.

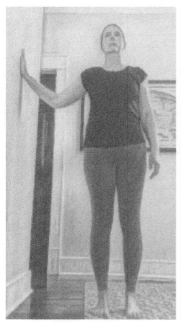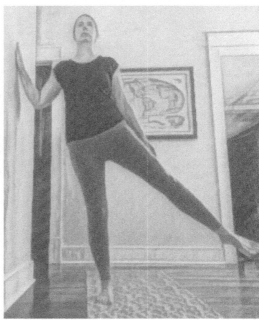

Wall Calf Raises with Hold: Stand facing a wall with your feet hip-width apart and your hands lightly resting on the wall for balance. Lift both heels off the ground as high as you can, coming onto the balls of your feet. Hold this raised position for a few seconds, feeling the contraction in your calf muscles. Lower your heels back down to the ground with control. Repeat for 3 sets of 15 repetitions.

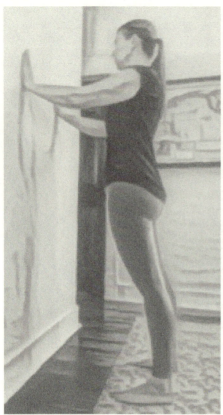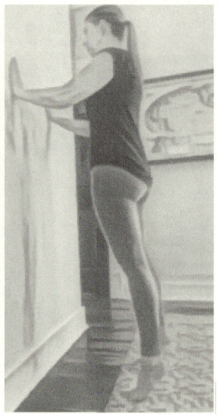

Wall Bridge with Leg Extension: Lie on your back with your hips close to a wall, your knees bent, and feet flat on the floor. Press your feet into the wall and lift your hips off the floor, coming into a bridge position. Keep your shoulders and upper back on the floor and engage your core and glutes to support your body. Extend one leg straight up towards the ceiling, keeping it aligned with your hip. Hold this position for a few seconds, then lower your leg back down. Repeat for 2 sets of 10 repetitions.

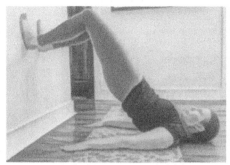 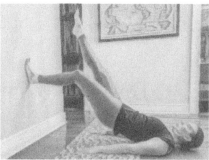

Day 18 - Balance and Stability

- Wall Roll-Down to Single-Leg Balance: 5 repetitions each leg
- Wall Single-Leg Squats with Rotation: 3 sets of 8 repetitions each leg
- Wall Plank with Arm and Leg Lift: 3 sets of 8 repetitions each side
- Wall Side Plank with Leg Lift: 3 sets of 8 repetitions each side
- Wall Leg Swings with Twist: 2 sets of 10 repetitions each leg

Wall Roll-Down to Single-Leg Balance: Stand with your back against the wall, feet about 5 inches from the wall and hip-width apart. Slowly roll down through your spine, feeling each vertebra pull away from the wall until your head, shoulders and spine are parallel to the floor. Walk your hands forward until you are in a plank position with your hands directly under your shoulders. Step one foot forward between your hands into a lunge position. Lift your back foot off the ground and extend it straight back, coming into a single-leg balance position. Hold the balance for a few seconds, then return your back foot to the ground. Walk your hands back towards your feet and slowly roll back up to standing against the wall, one vertebra at a time. Repeat the movement, alternating legs for each single-leg balance for 5 repetitions on each leg.

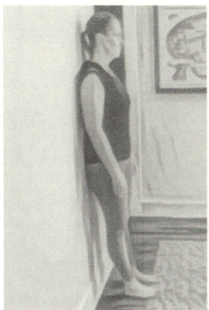
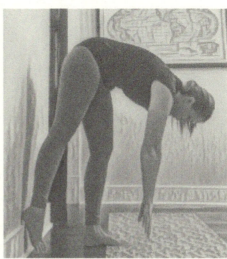

Wall Single-Leg Squats with Rotation: Stand with your back against a wall and your feet hip-width apart. Lift one foot off the ground and extend it straight out in front of you. Engage your core and lower into a squat on your standing leg, keeping your back flat against the wall. As you squat down, rotate your torso towards the lifted leg, bringing your opposite elbow towards your knee. Keep your chest lifted and your spine long throughout the movement. Push through your standing heel to return to the starting position. Repeat the squat with rotation on the same leg for the desired number of repetitions before switching to the other leg. Do 3 sets of 8 on each leg.

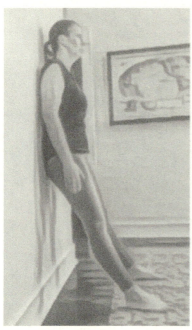
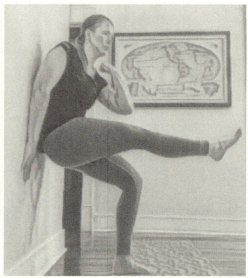

Wall Plank with Arm and Leg Lift: Start in a plank position facing away from the wall, with your hands on the floor directly under your shoulders and your feet resting against the wall. Engage your core and lift one arm off the ground, reaching it straight out in front of you. At the same time, lift the opposite leg off the ground, extending it straight out behind you. Hold the lifted arm and leg for a few seconds, then lower them back down. Repeat the movement with the opposite arm and leg. Continue alternating sides for 3 sets of 8 repetitions on each side.

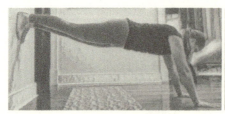
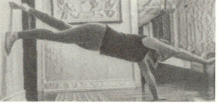

Wall Leg Swings with Twist: Stand sideways to the wall with one hand lightly resting on the wall for balance. Swing your leg forward and backward in a controlled motion, keeping it straight. As you swing your leg forward, rotate your torso towards the wall, reaching your opposite hand towards your swinging leg. Swing your leg backward while rotating your torso back to the starting position. Continue swinging your leg while rotating your torso, focusing on the twisting motion through your core. Do 2 sets of 10 on each leg.

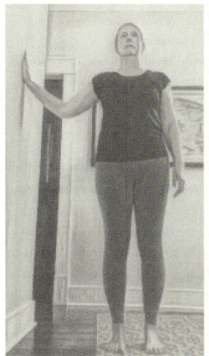 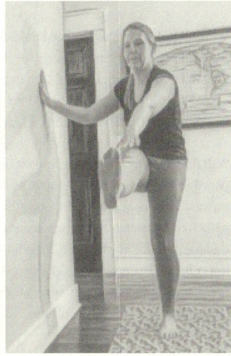

Day 19 - Flow

- Wall Roll-Down to Forward Fold: 5 repetitions
- Wall Hamstring Stretch with Toe Reach: Hold for 30 seconds each leg
- Wall Chest Opener with Backbend: Hold for 30 seconds
- Wall Quadriceps Stretch: Hold for 30 seconds each leg
- Wall Spinal Twist Stretch: Hold for 30 seconds each side

Wall Roll-Down to Forward Fold: Stand with your back against a wall and your feet hip-width apart. Slowly roll down through your spine, bending forward until your hands can touch the floor. Allow your head and arms to hang freely towards the floor, relaxing into the stretch. Hold the forward fold position for 20-30 seconds, feeling the stretch in your hamstrings and lower back. To come out of the stretch, slowly roll back up through your spine, stacking each vertebra one on top of the other until you are standing tall again. Repeat for 5 repetitions.

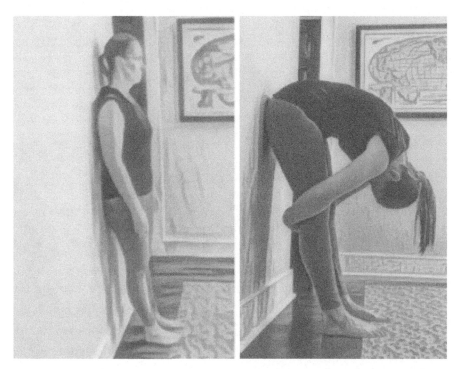

Wall Hamstring Stretch with Toe Reach: Lie on your back with your hips close to a wall and your legs extended upward, pressing against the wall. Keep your legs straight and flex your feet towards you. Slowly slide one leg down the wall, keeping it straight, until you feel a stretch in the back of your thigh (hamstring). Reach towards your toes with your hands, gently pulling your leg closer to your body to deepen the stretch. Hold the stretch for 30 seconds, then switch legs and repeat on the other side.

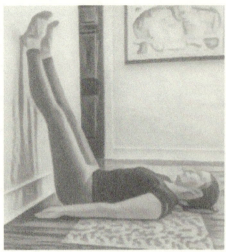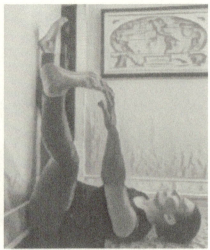

Wall Chest Opener with Back Bend: Stand facing a wall with your feet hip-width apart. Place your hands flat against the wall at shoulder height and slightly wider than shoulder width apart. Lean your body forward slightly, keeping your arms straight. Gently arch your back, allowing your chest to open towards the ceiling. Hold the back bend position for 30 seconds, feeling the stretch across your chest and front shoulder muscles. To come out of the stretch, slowly release the back bend and return to a neutral standing position.

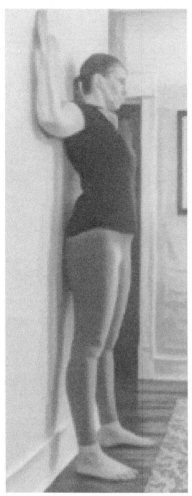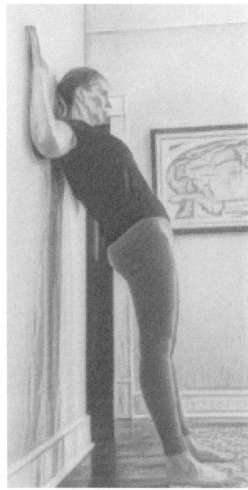

Wall Quadriceps Stretch: Stand facing away from a wall and place one hand lightly on the wall for balance. Bend one knee and bring your heel towards your buttocks, grasping your ankle with your free hand. Gently pull your heel towards your buttocks until you feel a stretch in the front of your thigh (quadriceps). Keep your knees close together and your torso upright. Hold the stretch for 30 seconds, then switch legs and repeat on the other side.

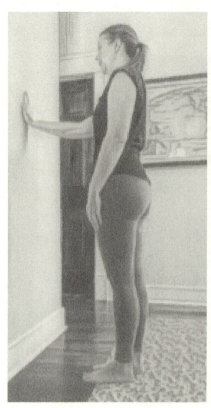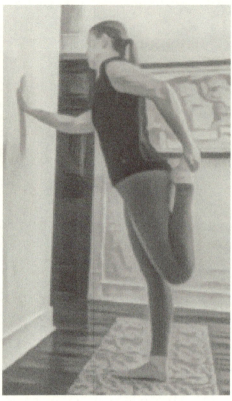

Wall Spinal Twist Stretch: Sit on the floor with your right side close to a wall. Lie on your back and swing your legs up against the wall, so your body forms an "L" shape, with your hips close to the wall and your legs extended vertically. Extend your arms out to the sides in a T-position, palms facing up. Lower both legs to the right side, allowing them to rest against the wall. Turn your head to the left and gaze in the opposite direction of your legs. Feel the stretch along your spine and through your chest and shoulders. Hold the stretch for 30 seconds, then return to the starting position and repeat on the other side.

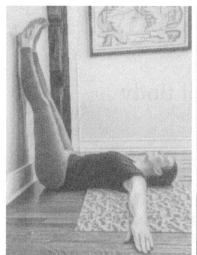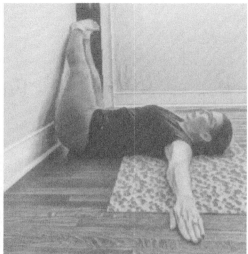

Day 20 - Full Body

- Wall Roll-Down to Plank: 5 repetitions
- Wall Squat to Overhead Reach with Rotation: 3 sets of 10 repetitions
- Wall Bridge with Leg Swings: 3 sets of 10 repetitions each leg
- Wall Plank to Side Plank: 3 sets of 8 repetitions each side
- Wall Roll-Up with Twist: 2 sets of 12 repetitions

Wall Roll-Down to Plank: Stand with your back against a wall and your feet hip-width apart. Slowly roll down through your spine, bending forward until your hands can touch the floor. Walk your hands forward until you are in a plank position with your hands directly under your shoulders. Engage your core to maintain a straight line from head to heels. Hold the plank position for a few seconds, focusing on stability and control. To return to the starting position, walk your hands back towards your feet and slowly roll back up to standing against the wall, one vertebra at a time. Repeat this for 5 repetitions.

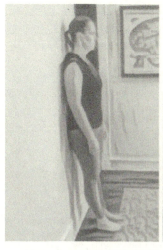
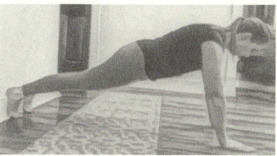

Wall Squat to Overhead Reach with Rotation: Stand with your back against a wall and your feet hip-width apart. Lower into a squat position by bending your knees and sliding your back down the wall until your thighs are parallel to the floor and your knees are at a 90-degree angle. Hold the squat position and extend your arms overhead. Rotate your torso to one side, reaching one arm towards the ceiling while keeping your hips square. Return to center and repeat the rotation on the opposite side. Continue alternating sides for 3 sets of 10 repetitions.

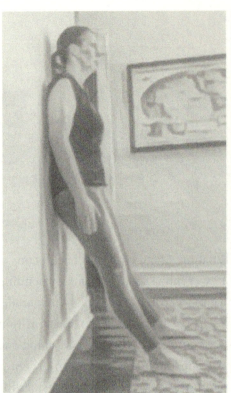 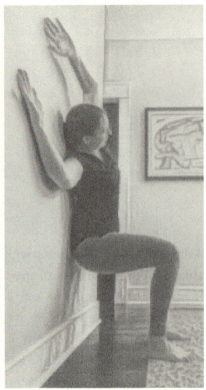

Wall Bridge with Leg Swings: Lie on your back with your hips close to a wall and your knees bent, feet flat on the floor. Press your feet into the wall and lift your hips off the floor, coming into a bridge position. Keep your shoulders and upper back on the floor and engage your core and glutes to support your body. Swing one leg out to the side as far as you can, then swing it back towards the center. Repeat the leg swings on the same side for the desired number of repetitions before switching to the other leg. Do this for 3 sets of 10 repetitions on each side.

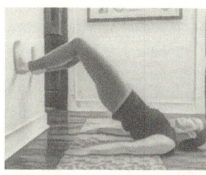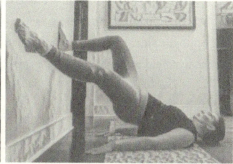

Wall Plank to Side Plank: Start in a plank position facing away from the wall, with your hands on the floor directly under your shoulders and your feet resting against the wall. Engage your core and lift one arm off the ground, rotating your torso to one side. Stack your feet and hips on top of each other to come into a side plank position, balancing on one hand and the side of one foot. Hold the side plank position for a few seconds, then return to the plank position. Repeat the movement, this time rotating to the opposite side. Continue alternating between plank and side plank for 3 sets of 8 repetitions on each side.

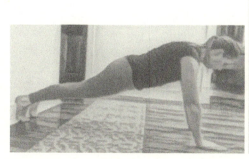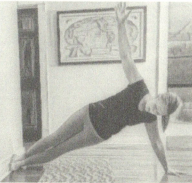

Wall Roll-Up with Twist: Start by lying on your back with your arms extended overhead and your legs straight, feet against the wall. Engage your core and slowly roll up through your spine, lifting your head, shoulders, and arms off the floor. Once you are sitting up tall, rotate your torso to one side, reaching your arms towards your foot. Return to center and slowly roll back down to the starting position, one vertebra at a time. Repeat the roll-up with twist on the opposite side, reaching the other arm towards the opposite foot. Continue alternating sides for 2 sets of 12 repetitions.

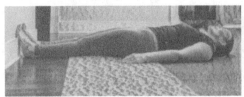 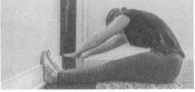

Day 21 - Recovery

Today choose a light activity such as walking, or stretching to promote recovery and prepare for the upcoming week. Focus your attention on unwinding and revitalizing your body and mind.

Day 22 - Core Strength

- Wall Roll-Down to Twist: 5 repetitions each side
- Wall Plank with Knee to Opposite Elbow: 3 sets of 10 repetitions each side
- Wall Pike to Pike Push-Up: 3 sets of 8 repetitions
- Wall Side Plank with Leg Lift and Reach: 3 sets of 8 repetitions each side
- Wall Bicycle Crunches: 2 sets of 15 repetitions each side

Wall Roll-Down to Twist: Start by standing tall with your back against a wall and your feet hip-width apart. Engage your core and slowly roll down through your spine, bending forward until your hands can touch the floor. Once your hands are on the floor, walk them out in front of you until you are in a plank position with your hands directly under your shoulders. Rotate your torso to one side, lifting one arm towards the ceiling while keeping your hips square. Hold the twist for a moment, feeling the stretch through your spine and oblique muscles. Return to plank position and repeat the twist on the opposite side. Walk your hands back towards your feet and slowly roll back up to standing against the wall, one vertebra at a time. Do 5 repetitions on each side.

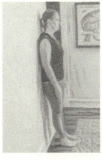
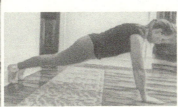
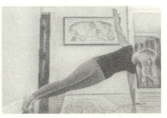

Wall Plank with Knee to Opposite Elbow: Start in a plank position facing away from the wall, with your hands on the floor directly under your shoulders and your feet resting against the wall. Engage your core and lift one foot off the wall, bringing your knee towards the opposite elbow. Hold the knee-to-elbow position for a moment, feeling the contraction in your oblique muscles. Return your foot to the wall and repeat the movement with the opposite knee and elbow. Continue alternating sides for 3 sets of 10 repetitions on each side.

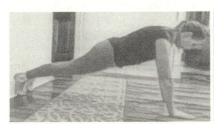
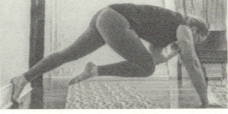

Wall Pike to Pike Push-Up: Start in a plank position facing away from the wall, with your hands on the floor directly under your shoulders and your feet resting against the wall. Engage your core, lift your hips towards the ceiling, and pull your feet away from the wall coming into a pike position with your body forming an inverted "V". Bend your elbows to lower your head towards the floor, performing a pike push-up. Push through your palms to press back up to the starting position. Continue with the pike push-ups for 3 sets of 8 repetitions.

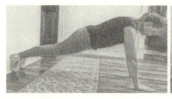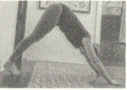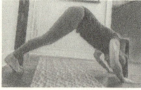

Wall Side Plank with Leg Lift and Reach: Start in a side plank position facing the wall, with your forearm on the floor and your feet stacked. Engage your core and lift your top leg towards the ceiling, keeping it straight. At the same time, reach your top arm overhead, feeling the stretch through your side body. Hold the leg lift and reach for a moment, then return to the starting position. Repeat the movement for 3 sets of 8 on each side.

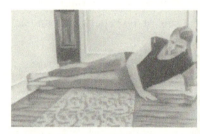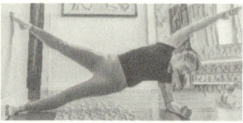

Wall Bicycle Crunches: Lie on your back with your hips close to a wall and your legs extended upward, pressing against the wall. Place your hands lightly behind your head, elbows pointing out to the sides. Engage your core and lift your shoulder blades off the floor, bringing your chest towards your knees. Bring one knee towards your chest while simultaneously rotating your torso to bring the opposite elbow towards the knee. Straighten the bent leg as you switch sides, bringing the other knee towards your chest while rotating your torso to bring the opposite elbow towards the knee. Continue alternating sides in a pedaling motion, focusing on the rotation through your torso. Repeat the exercise for 2 sets of 15 repetitions on each side.

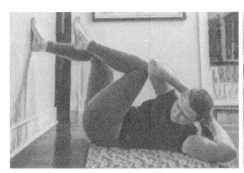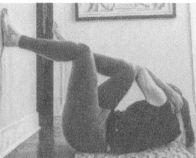

Day 23 - Upper Body

- Wall Roll-Down to Push-Up: 5 repetitions
- Wall Push-Ups with Shoulder Tap: 3 sets of 10 repetitions
- Wall Tricep Dips with Leg Extension: 3 sets of 10 repetitions
- Wall Arm Circles: 3 sets of 15 repetitions forward and backward
- Wall Plank with Alternating Arm Reach: 2 sets of 12 repetitions each side

Wall Roll-Down to Push-Up: Start by standing tall with your back against a wall and your feet hip-width apart. Engage your core and slowly roll down through your spine, bending forward until your hands can touch the floor. Once your hands are on the floor, walk them out in front of you until you are in a plank position with your hands directly under your shoulders. Do one push-up and then walk your hands back towards your feet and slowly roll back up to standing against the wall, one vertebra at a time. Repeat the movement for 5 repetitions.

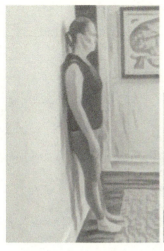
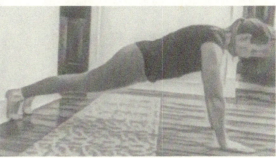

Wall Push-Ups with Shoulder Tap: Stand facing a wall and place your hands on the wall slightly wider than shoulder-width apart, at chest height and take a step back. Engage your core and bend your elbows to lower your chest towards the wall, performing a push-up. Push through your palms to return to the starting position, then tap one hand to the opposite shoulder. Repeat the push-up, then tap the other hand to the opposite shoulder. Continue alternating shoulder taps for 3 sets of 10 repetitions. You may try this while holding a resistance band for more difficulty.

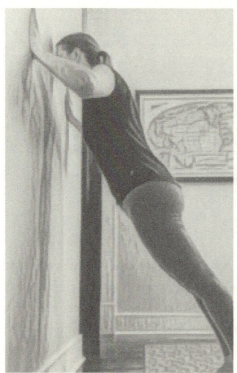
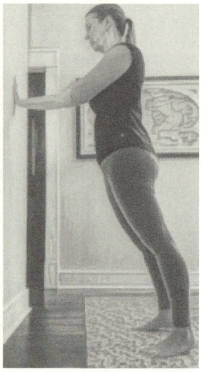

Wall Tricep Dips with Leg Extension: Sit on the floor with your back against the wall, knees bent, and feet flat on the floor. Place your hands on the wall behind your hips, fingers pointing towards your feet. Press through your palms to lift your hips off the floor, straightening your arms. Lower your hips towards the floor by bending your elbows, keeping them close to your body. Push through your palms to return to the starting position, simultaneously extending one leg straight out in front of you. Lower your leg back to the floor and repeat the tricep dip with the opposite leg extended. Continue alternating leg extensions with tricep dips 3 sets of 10 repetitions.

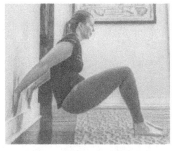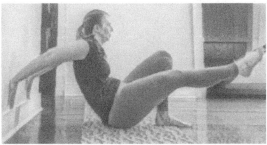

Wall Arm Circles: Stand facing the wall with your arms extended out toward the wall at shoulder height, pressing your palms flat against the wall. Begin making circular motions with your arms, moving them forward in small circles. Gradually increase the size of the circles, keeping your arms straight and shoulders relaxed. After completing forward circles, reverse the direction and perform circles in the opposite direction. Repeat 3 sets of 15 forward and backward. Try this with a resistance band keeping it tight from one hand around your back to the other hand for more difficulty.

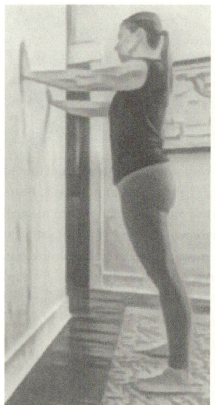 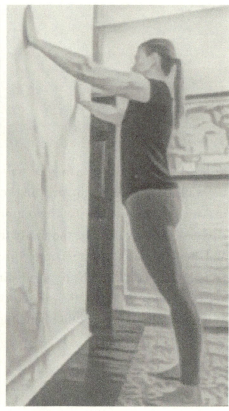

Wall Plank with Alternating Arm Reach: Start in a plank position facing away from the wall, with your hands on the floor directly under your shoulders and your feet resting against the wall. Engage your core and lift one hand off the floor, reaching it straight out in front of you. Hold the arm reach for a moment, then return the hand to the floor and switch sides. Continue alternating arm reaches for 2 sets of 12 repetitions on each side. Try this with a resistance band.

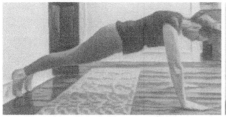 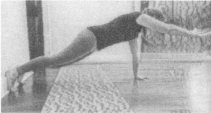

Day 24 - Lower Body

- Wall Roll-Down to Reverse Lunge: 5 repetitions each leg
- Wall Squats with Pulse and Hold: 3 sets of 12 repetitions
- Wall Side Leg Lifts: 3 sets of 12 repetitions each leg
- Wall Calf Raises: 3 sets of 20 repetitions
- Wall Bridge with Leg Extension: 2 sets of 12 repetitions each leg

Wall Roll-Down to Reverse Lunge: Stand tall with your back against a wall and your feet hip-width apart. Engage your core and slowly roll down through your spine, bending forward until your hands can touch the floor. Once your hands are on the floor, walk them out in front of you until you are in a plank position with your hands directly under your shoulders. Step one foot forward between your hands into a reverse lunge position. Lower your back knee towards the floor until both knees are bent at 90-degree angles. Push through your front heel to return to standing, then step your foot back to plank position. Walk your hands back towards your feet and slowly roll back up to standing against the wall, one vertebra at a time. Repeat the movement, alternating legs for each reverse lunge. Do 5 repetitions on each side.

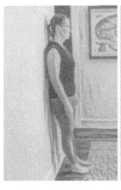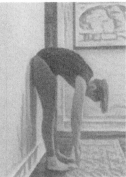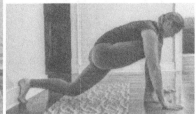

Wall Squats with Pulse and Hold: Stand with your back against a wall and your feet hip-width apart. Place a resistance band just above your knees and loop it around your thighs. Lower into a squat position by bending your knees and sliding your back down the wall until your thighs are parallel to the floor and your knees are at a 90-degree angle. Hold the squat position and pulse up and down slightly, moving only a few inches. After pulsing, hold the squat position for 5-10 seconds, feeling the burn in your quadriceps and glutes. Push through your heels to return to standing and repeat the movement for 3 sets of 12 repetitions.

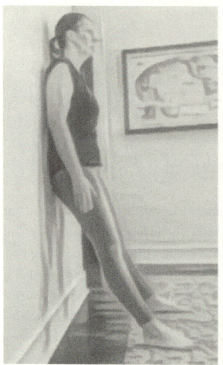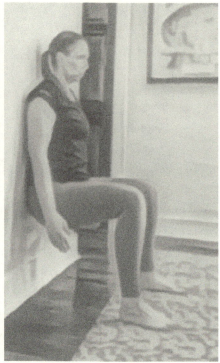

Wall Side Leg Lifts: Stand sideways to a wall with one hand lightly resting on the wall for balance. Lift your outside leg out to the side as high as you can keeping it straight. Lower your leg back down to the starting position with control. Repeat the movement for the desired number of repetitions on one side before switching to the other side. Keep your torso stable and avoid leaning towards the wall. Do 3 sets of 12 on each side. For more difficulty, try this with a resistance band around your ankles or thighs.

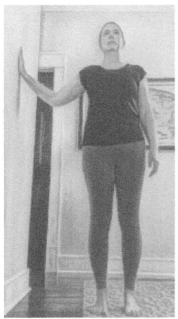 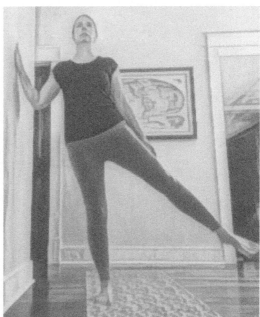

Wall Calf Raises: Stand facing a wall with your feet hip-width apart. Hold onto the wall for balance if needed. Lift your heels off the ground as high as you can, coming onto the balls of your feet. Hold the raised position for a moment, then lower your heels back down towards the floor. Repeat the calf raises for 3 sets of 20 repetitions. Try this with weights or a resistance band for more difficulty.

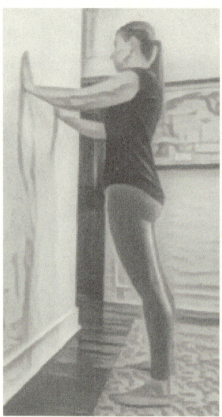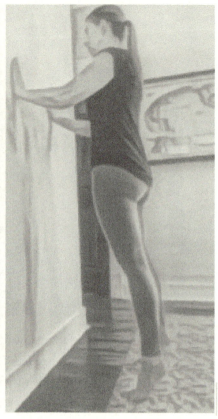

Wall Bridge with Leg Extension: Lie on your back with your hips close to a wall and your knees bent, feet flat on the floor. Press your feet into the wall and lift your hips off the floor, coming into a bridge position. Keep your shoulders and upper back on the floor and engage your core and glutes to support your body. Extend one leg straight up towards the ceiling. Hold this position for a few seconds, then lower your leg back down. Repeat the leg extension on the same side for the desired number of repetitions before switching to the other leg. Do 2 sets of 12 on each leg. This can be done with a resistance band around your thighs for more difficulty.

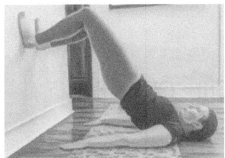 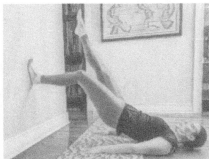

Day 25 - Stability Challenge

- Wall Roll-Down to Single-Leg Balance with Arm Circles: 5 repetitions each leg
- Wall Single-Leg Squats: 3 sets of 8 repetitions each leg
- Wall Plank with Arm and Leg Lift and Rotation: 3 sets of 8 repetitions each side
- Wall Side Plank with Leg Lift and Hip Dip: 3 sets of 8 repetitions each side
- Wall Leg Swings: 2 sets of 10 repetitions each leg

Wall Roll-Down to Single-Leg Balance with Arm Circles: Stand tall with your back against a wall and your feet hip-width apart. Engage your core and slowly roll down through your spine, bending forward until your hands can touch the floor. Once your hands are on the floor, walk them out in front of you until you are in a plank position with your hands directly under your shoulders. Shift your weight onto one foot and lift the opposite foot off the floor, coming into a single-leg balance position. While balancing on one leg, make small circles with your arms, moving them forward in a controlled motion. If you have trouble sliding your hands, try one at a time. After completing the circles, reverse the motion and make circles in the opposite direction. Hold the single-leg balance with arm circles for a few seconds, then return your foot to the floor and repeat on the opposite side. Do 5 repetitions on each leg.

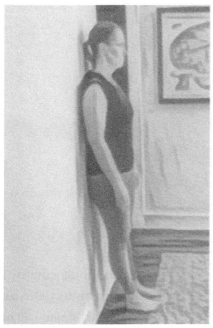
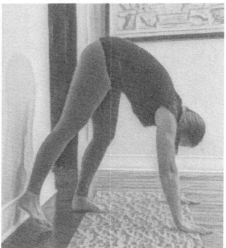

Wall Single-Leg Squats: Stand facing away from a wall and place one hand lightly on the wall for balance. Lift one foot off the floor and extend it straight out in front of you. Engage your core and bend your standing knee, lowering your body into a single-leg squat Keep your chest lifted and your spine straight throughout the movement. Push through your standing heel to return to the starting position. Repeat the single-leg squat for the desired number of repetitions on one leg before switching to the other leg. Do 3 sets of 8 on each leg.

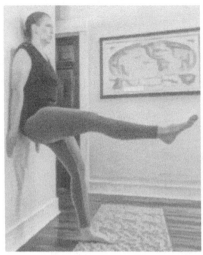
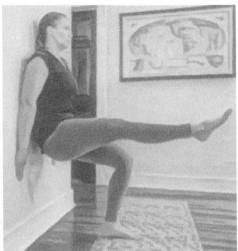

Wall Plank with Arm and Rotation: Start in a plank position facing away from the wall, with your hands on the floor directly under your shoulders and your feet resting against the wall. Engage your core and lift one arm off the ground, rotating your torso to one side and reaching the arm towards the ceiling. Hold the lifted arm for a few seconds, then return them to the starting position. Repeat the movement with the opposite arm, rotating to the other side. Continue alternating arm lifts with rotation for 3 sets of 8 repetitions on each side.

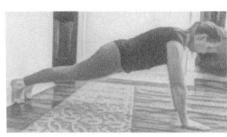
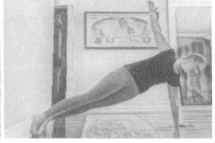

Wall Side Plank with Leg Lift and Hip Dip: Start in a side plank position facing the wall, with your forearm on the floor and your feet stacked. Engage your core and lift your top leg towards the ceiling, keeping it straight. At the same time, lower your hips towards the floor, performing a hip dip. Lift your hips back up to the starting position and lower your leg back down. Repeat the leg lift and hip dip for the desired number of repetitions on one side before switching to the other side. Do 3 sets of 8 repetitions on each side. This can be done with a resistance band around your thighs for more difficulty.

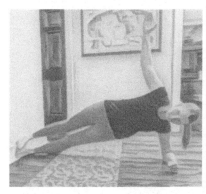 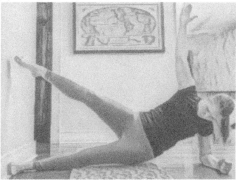

Wall Leg Swings: Stand sideways to a wall with one hand lightly resting on the wall for balance. Swing your outside leg forward and backward in a controlled motion, keeping it straight. After completing the desired number of swings, switch sides and repeat with the other leg. Do 2 sets of 10 on each leg. Try this with a resistance band for more difficulty.

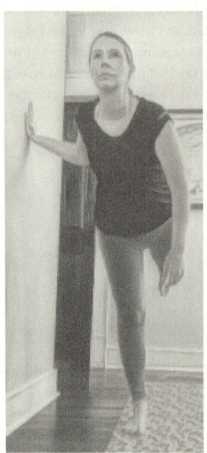
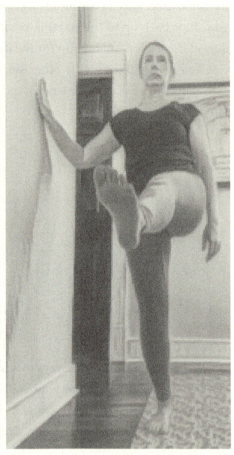

Day 26 - Flexibility and Strength

- Wall Roll-Down to Forward Fold Stretch: 5 repetitions
- Wall Hamstring Stretch with Leg Lift: Hold for 30 seconds each leg
- Wall Chest Opener with Backbend: Hold for 30 seconds
- Wall Quadriceps Stretch with Hip Flexor Activation: Hold for 30 seconds each leg
- Wall Spinal Twist Stretch: Hold for 30 seconds each side

Wall Roll-Down to Forward Fold Stretch: Stand tall with your back against a wall and your feet hip-width apart. Engage your core and slowly roll down through your spine, bending forward until your hands can touch the floor. Once your hands are on the floor, walk them out in front of you until you feel a stretch in your hamstrings. Hold the stretch for 30 seconds, then slowly roll back up to standing against the wall, one vertebra at a time. Repeat 5 times.

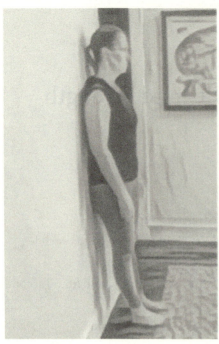
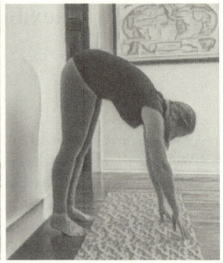

Wall Hamstring Stretch with Leg Lift: Lie on your back with your hips close to a wall and your legs extended upward, pressing against the wall. Use your hands to gently pull one leg towards your chest, feeling the stretch in your hamstring. Lift your other leg towards the ceiling, keeping it straight and pressing against the wall. Hold the stretch for 30 seconds, then switch legs and repeat on the other side.

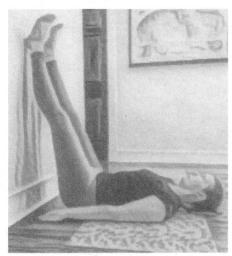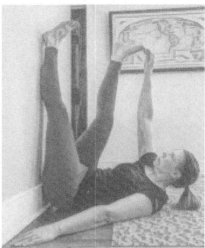

Wall Chest Opener with Back Bend: Stand facing a wall with your feet hip-width apart. Step forward with one foot and place your hands on the wall, slightly wider than shoulder-width apart. Lean forward slightly, keeping your arms straight, and allow your chest to open towards the wall. Engage your core and gently arch your back, pressing your chest forward and lifting your gaze towards the ceiling. Hold the back bend position for 30 seconds, then release and return to standing.

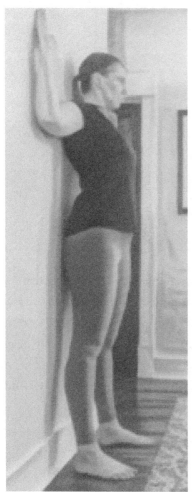 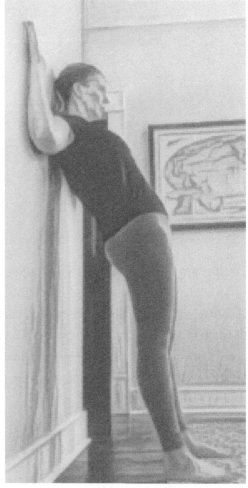

Wall Quadriceps Stretch with Hip Flexor Activation: Stand facing away from a wall with your feet hip-width apart. Place one hand on the wall for balance if needed. Bend one knee and bring your heel towards your buttocks, grasping your ankle with your hand. Engage your core and press your hips forward slightly to activate your hip flexors while maintaining the stretch in your quadriceps. Hold the stretch for 30 seconds, then switch legs and repeat on the other side.

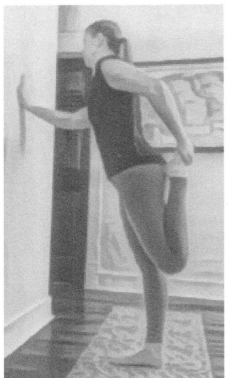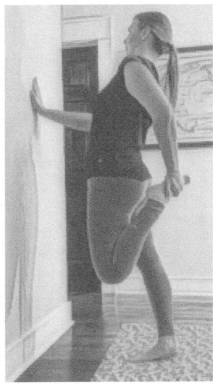

Wall Spinal Twist Stretch: Sit on the floor with your right side close to a wall. Lie on your back and swing your legs up against the wall, so your body forms an "L" shape, with your hips close to the wall and your legs extended vertically. Hold your arms out to the sides in a T-position for support. Lower both legs to one side, allowing them to rest against the wall. Engage your core and gently rotate your torso in the opposite direction, feeling the stretch through your spine and chest. Hold the stretch for 30 seconds, then return to the starting position and repeat on the other side.

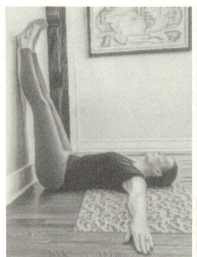 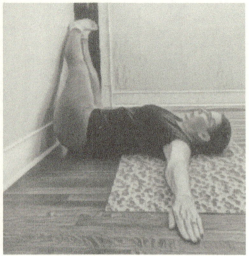

Day 27 - Full Body

- Wall Roll-Down to Plank with Leg Lift: 5 repetitions
- Wall Squat to Overhead Reach: 3 sets of 10 repetitions
- Wall Bridge with Leg Swings: 3 sets of 10 repetitions each leg
- Wall Plank to Side Plank with Arm Reach: 3 sets of 8 repetitions each side
- Wall Roll-Up to Twist: 2 sets of 12 repetitions

Wall Roll-Down to Plank with Leg Lift: Stand tall with your back against a wall and your feet hip-width apart. Engage your core and slowly roll down through your spine, bending forward until your hands can touch the floor. Once your hands are on the floor, walk them out in front of you until you are in a plank position with your hands directly under your shoulders. Engage your core and lift one leg up off the ground, extending it straight out behind you. Hold the leg lift for a moment, then lower your leg back to the ground. Repeat the leg lift on the opposite side, alternating legs for 5 repetitions. This can be done with a resistance band around your thighs.

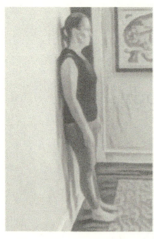
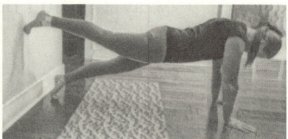

Wall Squat to Overhead Reach with Rotation: Stand with your back against a wall and your feet hip-width apart. Lower into a squat position by bending your knees and sliding your back down the wall until your thighs are parallel to the floor and your knees are at a 90-degree angle. Hold the squat position and rotate your torso to one side, reaching one arm towards the ceiling while keeping your hips square. Return to center and repeat the rotation on the opposite side. Continue alternating sides for 3 sets of 10 repetitions.

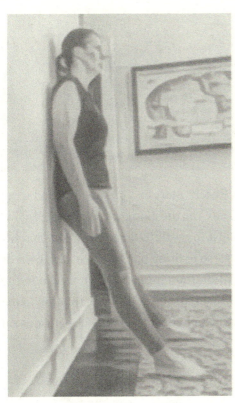 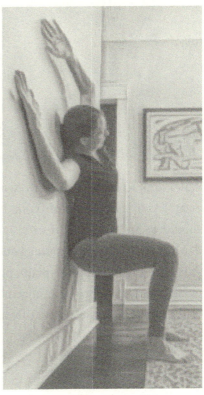

Wall Bridge with Leg Swings: Lie on your back with your hips close to a wall and your knees bent, feet flat on the floor. Press your feet into the wall and lift your hips off the floor, coming into a bridge position. Keep your shoulders and upper back on the floor and engage your core and glutes to support your body. Swing one leg out to the side as far as you can, then swing it back towards the center. Repeat the leg swings on the same side for the desired number of repetitions before switching to the other leg. Do 3 sets of 10 on each side. Try this with a resistance band for more difficulty.

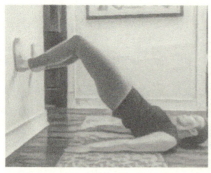
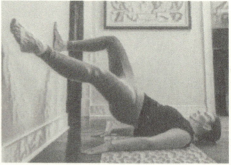

Wall Plank to Side Plank with Arm Reach: Start in a plank position facing away from the wall, with your hands on the floor directly under your shoulders and your feet resting against the wall. Engage your core and lift one hand off floor, rotating your torso to bring the extended arm towards the ceiling. Hold the side plank position for a moment, then return to the plank position. Repeat the movement with the opposite arm, rotating to the other side. Continue alternating arm reaches for 3 sets of 8 repetitions on each side.

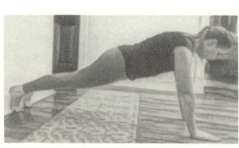
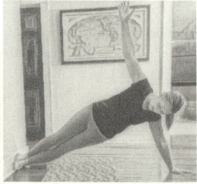

Wall Roll-Up to Twist: Start by lying on your back with your arms extended overhead and your legs straight, feet against the wall. Engage your core and slowly roll up through your spine, lifting your head, shoulders, and arms off the floor. Once you are sitting up tall, rotate your torso to one side, reaching one arm towards the opposite foot. Return to center and slowly roll back down to the starting position, one vertebra at a time. Repeat the roll-up with twist on the opposite side, reaching the other arm towards the opposite foot. Continue alternating sides for 2 sets of 12 repetitions.

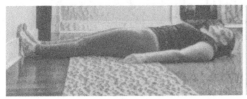 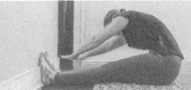

Day 28 - Celebrate Your Progress

Stretch or go for a walk to give your body time to heal. Consider how far your adventure has brought you. Compare how you have changed, mentally and physically, using your journal, measurements, and the photos you took before you started. Above all, acknowledge your accomplishments and schedule future steps in your quest for health and fitness!

If you feel this book was helpful to you in any way, please take the time to leave me a review!

Resources

OpenAI. (2024). ChatGPT (3.5) [Large language model]. https://chat.openai.
com

Made in the USA
Coppell, TX
11 May 2024

32267399R10083